SELEN

Research has found that there is a link between low selenium levels in our bodies and many of today's diseases. Dr Eric Trimmer tells the story and explains how we can be sure to get sufficient of this vital trace element to stay healthy.

By the same author
THE MAGIC OF MAGNESIUM

Selenium

The trace element for health
and life extension

by

Dr Eric Trimmer

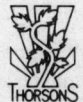

THORSONS PUBLISHING GROUP

First published 1988

© ERIC TRIMMER 1988

All rights reserved. No part of this book may be reproduced or utilized in any form or by any means, electronic or mechanical, including photocopying, recording or by any information storage and retrieval system, without permission in writing from the Publisher.

British Library Cataloguing in Publication Data

Trimmer, Eric
Selenium: the trace element for health
and life extension.
1. Selenium in human nutrition
I. Title
613.2'8   TX553.S4

ISBN 0-7225-1388-7

*Published by Thorsons Publishers Limited,
Wellingborough, Northamptonshire, NN8 2RQ, England*

Printed in Great Britain by
Richard Clay Limited, Bungay, Suffolk

1 3 5 7 9 10 8 6 4 2

Contents

	Introduction	7
Chapter		
1.	What is selenium?	11
2.	What's wrong with testimonials?	18
3.	Trace elements and good health	23
4.	Medical geography and selenium	29
5.	Selenium and life extension	35
6.	Beating arthritis with selenium	41
7.	How selenium spares the heart	48
8.	Cancer prevention and selenium	56
9.	Escaping micronutrient failure	67
10.	Feeling one degree under — and selenium	75
11.	Not only but also	80
12.	Selenium as health insurance	88
	Index	94

NOTE TO READERS

Before following any self-help advice given in this book readers are earnestly urged to give careful consideration to the nature of their particular health problem, and to consult a competent physician if in any doubt. This book should not be regarded as a substitute for professional medical treatment, and whilst every care is taken to ensure the accuracy of the content, the author and the publishers cannot accept legal responsibility for any problem arising as a result of experimentation with the methods described.

Introduction

Five years ago Alan Lewis, now Executive Director of Britain's leading health magazine, *Here's Health,* told an amazing story. It was about selenium and a remarkable community living on the north Norfolk coast in East Anglia, England. Now I want to bring this story right up to date in the light of recent research.

Alan Lewis told us about Billy Collins and his wife, Amy. Billy was 96 and Amy was 91. The incredible thing about these folk was that although they were old in years they were extraordinarily young in heart, and they were fit and active. Alan had a theory about the reasons that lay behind this, but like all good medical journalists he is not the sort of man to accept a theory about health and longevity on its face value. So he started looking at facts and figures that might support or refute the theory that was forming in his mind. The results of extensive local investigations made him sit up and take notice even more.

The area in which his friends Billy and Amy were living claimed four active centenarians, all delighted with their telegrams from the Queen! The local church choir was unusual too — its average age was 73 — and the local horticultural association boasted a large number of gardeners with an average age of 70 plus. The very active Darby and Joan club in the area (average age 74) had had to close its doors to new members because it could not cope with the pressure for additional membership and had generated an embarrassingly long waiting list!

When I first read Alan's book I had reason to think about my youth in East Anglia. When I was a youngster my family used regularly to visit the area for our summer holidays. The people we used to lodge with there were a Mr and Mrs Perfect. They were perfect in many ways. He was the local cobbler and still worked in his shop repairing shoes in his late 70s with a degree of energy and excellence that would have been the envy of many a younger man. His wife, of around the same age,

Mortality among males from coronary heart disease (by regional health authorities), in England, Wales and Scotland, 1979, rates per 1,000 population.

	Age group		
Region	45-54	55-64	65-74
England	2.72	7.18	16.05
Regions:			
Northern	3.31	8.98	17.93
Yorkshire	3.12	8.04	18.42
Trent	2.87	7.44	16.55
East Anglia	2.07	5.75	14.47
NW Thames	2.44	6.42	14.22
NE Thames	2.52	6.96	15.00
SE Thames	2.35	6.63	14.93
SW Thames	2.26	5.90	14.08
Wessex	2.52	6.68	16.09
Oxford	2.17	5.65	14.14
South Western	2.45	6.96	16.14
West Midlands	2.76	7.05	15.68
Mersey	3.27	8.25	16.94
North Western	3.37	8.49	18.70
Wales	3.05	8.12	18.43
Scotland	3.65	9.12	19.82
Excess of highest rate over lowest	76 per cent	61 per cent	41 per cent

Source Office of Population Censuses and Surveys

East Anglia has the lowest mortality from coronary heart disease. It also enjoys the highest soil selenium levels.

used to run the little boarding house we lodged in and was a fine cook and marvellous housewife. The youngest of their large family who still lived with them, Cliff, was a 'mere boy' in his late 50s, and he used to take my father and I out night-fishing — after working a long day for a local farmer. The summer's day started at 5.30 a.m. for him and yet when we returned with a couple of buckets full of sea bass at around 10 p.m. every night — a fair proportion of which appeared on our lunch table next day — he was as fresh as a daisy!

The answer is in the soil

Since most of the studies show that long-lived folk are usually closely involved with the land and live off local produce, the secret must surely lie in the soil and the sea. We have known for some time that people living and working in agricultural communities, and who feed themselves off the food they grow locally, tend to live longer and keep fitter than city dwellers who live on more sophisticated produce.

The fertile valleys of the Andes, for instance, produce an abundance of food and a distinct tendency towards a long and active life for the people living there. Exactly what is it that produces this unexpected health bonus? My own researches into the question started over 20 years ago when I was writing a book entitled *The History of Rejuvenation* (Robert Hale, 1967). Painstakingly I examined a great many substances that had been used traditionally in the search for a longer and healthier life and which had proved their worth by long and successful usage. At the time I found the vast variation in these favoured remedies quite baffling. For instance, the ancient Greeks thought highly of dishes containing mussels, crabs, snails and eggs for this purpose, especially when they were cooked with mushrooms and garlic. Another favourite from ancient times was the plant called mandrake — a native of the rocky areas of Spain, Sicily, Crete, Syria and North Africa, whose forked root dives down into rock crevices for sustenance.

Mandrake is even described in the Old Testament of the Bible when Rachel welcomes the sight of mandrakes, gathered by Leah as a suitable rejuvenant for her husband Jacob.

Then again old herbals compiled in Britain and Europe from the Middle Ages onwards often sing the praises of the roots of the purple orchid, which then grew widely, as a powerful rejuvenating substance. In no way was this a 'five-day wonder' type of health craze because 300 years later, in the eighteenth century, orchids were still widely grown for the manufacture of a health-giving drink called Salep, much praised for its restorative properties.

At other times and in other places other plants have gained favour among citizens of both sexes who wanted to 'live long and die young'. For example the roots of sea holly, widely grown in East Anglia, were 'candied' and sold as Colchester Comfits and their preparation was described in great detail by the famous herbalist Gerard.

Secrets from nature

It has always seemed to me a good indication that there *is* 'something in' a remedy for this or that when we see generations of farmers and animal husbanders routinely giving it to cattle and horses to improve their animals' general condition. One such health-giving substance praised and used by farmers from shores as far apart as those of India and Africa is fenugreek. When this two-foot high annual herb with its cherry red flowers is added to fodder, the condition of the cattle improves enormously.

For years it has been tempting to shrug this sort of thing off as yet another fanciful finding of the *Green Medicine* buffs. Now we know that *Faenum graecum* has a rich vitamin and mineral content and thus the whole subject becomes more worthy of our consideration.

When I was writing *The History of Rejuvenation,* like most doctors and medical and nutritional researchers, I had not heard of selenium or other trace elements as being related to health to any great extent. In fact only a handful of quite specialized scientific personnel had come across selenium at this time. If evidence that became available to a handful of research workers in the late 1950s had been common knowledge when I was writing my book I might have linked selenium with yet another seemingly 'inexplicable' health fad that was prevalent throughout the whole of Europe and Great Britain from Roman times onward when people of every social class started to realize the health benefits of 'taking the waters'.

Slowly but inexorably it has become obvious that the drinking of certain spa waters provides interesting and effective health bonuses. And towns like Bath and Malvern, Epsom and Buxton in England were virtually put on the map as the first real health centres due to the minerals and trace elements their 'waters' contained.

Why rejuvenation happened

Looking back over many of the remarkable accounts of unusual and unexpected health improvements that have been faithfully recorded by careful people throughout the ages, and which have largely been ignored by scientific medicine simply because it could not explain them, it now seems likely that trace elements were the substances providing the 'magic' to a large number of the 'inexplicable' cures so favoured by our ancestors. And on reflection a large and unsuspected contribution to that magic was made by selenium.

CHAPTER 1
What is selenium?

Physically selenium is a pretty unimpressive steely grey metal with an atomic weight of 78.96 and a relative density of 4.81. But it does have one important and impressive physical characteristic, which has endeared it to the manufacturers of photo-electric cells for many years. It has the special property of conducting electricity but *only* when it is exposed to light.

Although such properties are hardly worth knowing about from the health point of view, and nobody could say they are likely to arouse a twinkle of interest in a doctor's eye, before we leave this dry side of selenium there are two other physical characteristics I would like to mention. We will come back to them later, for they are of more general interest and importance. Selenium melts at a temperature of 217°C (423°F) and vaporises quite quickly after that. But perhaps, from the health point of view, the most important thing about selenium is that it is not only a trace element, but among trace elements it is something quite special — it is an *ultra trace element*, i.e. a substance that is present in foodstuffs only in an incredibly small quantity. This is really extremely relevant, for a tiny trace of something is very easy to lose — and then you finish up with nothing!

What is a trace element?

When new terms evolve they often 'sound good' scientifically. But to the ordinary person they do not mean anything very tangible. You know and I know what a *trace* of something is. It is pretty small! But just *how* small is important because that 'trace' in some circumstances, as we shall see later, has an influence on whether you and I keep fit. This smallness factor may be 'visualized' in the following way. An ounce of something, be it flour or sugar, is easy enough to contemplate. Divide an ounce of sugar into 28 portions and each will weigh 1 gram. If you divide one of those little gram-sized heaps of sugar into a thousand tiny heaps, each little pile — a mere speck — will weigh a *milligram*. Here you have to stop real visualization and go into the world of your imagination, for next I want you to imagine dividing one of those specks into a further thousand 'pieces'. Now each would weigh a *microgram*. If a gram of a substance (A) contains just one microgram of another substance (B), another way of expressing this is to say that A contains one part per million of B in it.

Now we are getting near to appreciating what is meant by trace elements. If a gram of substance A contains only a thousandth of a part of a microgram of B in it then you can say that B is present in one part per billion, and that's the size of the 'trace' we are talking about as far as trace elements in food are concerned.

Can such miniscule traces be important? Well, all the recent evidence that has come to light in the last few years suggests that they *are* vital to health and well-being. One neat little analogy I came across recently illustrates the point quite well. Imagine a giant Boeing 747 air liner being fuelled up for a transatlantic flight — the amount of fuel necessary amounts to about 14,000 gallons. Of course, in practice the airline operator will always allow a wide safety margin and put in a few thousand extra gallons to be on the safe side. But theoretically only 14,000 gallons are necessary. If, however, you started with 14,000 gallons only and then reduced it by a few parts per billion (the odd pint or so) the plane would never make the trip! This gets as near as I can to a practical understanding of the trace element situation. We need them in very small quantities to make a safe trip through life — and we must not forget this. We are liable to crash rather unexpectedly if we take liberties with them.

Enter selenium

Selenium was really first 'discovered' in the trace element sense due to the work of one man. Like Martin Luther King he was 'a man with a dream'. The dream was to be remembered as having cured one disease. His name was Klaus Schwartz, and he realized his ambition as we shall see in Chapter 7. During the first half of this century the major nutritional breakthrough was undoubtedly the discovery of the vitamins. In fact during 1926 and 1948 vitamins A, B, C, D, E and K were all identified and isolated from the various foods that are their natural sources, and by the time the 1950s had arrived many nutritionists felt that to a large extent the relationship between bad health and bad diets was largely a matter of vitamins.

Here and there, however, there were nutritional scientists who were puzzling away at other dietary health problems. As long ago as the turn of the century doctors knew that two mineral substances, iron and iodine, were necessary for good health. If there was not enough iron in the diet people got anaemic. If there was not enough iodine they developed disfiguring goitres. Between 1928 and 1935 copper, manganese, zinc and cobalt were also recognized to be essential nutrients. But in 1957 after ten years of continuous research Klaus Schwartz, then a scientist at the National Institute of Health, identified selenium and showed that it was involved in a form of (deficiency) disease in rats.

This was really the starting point of the modern story of selenium and health. From then on our knowledge of this amazing substance, which was named after Selene, the goddess of the moon, progressed rapidly. To start with nobody could fathom how this element, measured in such minute traces, could have an effect on health, disease and ageing. Then in 1973 Dr J. T. Rotruck, of the University of Wisconsin, and his co-workers, identified selenium in a vital tissue enzyme called glutathione peroxidase. This enzyme holds a key position in the basic integrity of all healthy cell chemistry. If our body intake and absorption of selenium drops below certain vital levels we cannot make enough of this enzyme for our cells to function effectively, and the various manifestations of selenium deficiency outlined in this book are liable to develop.

Who is short of selenium?

In the United Kingdom almost everybody tends to be short of selenium, and we will return to this in detail later. Although nutritional science had a basic knowledge of selenium, the general public did not really start hearing about it until the beginning of this decade when Richard Passwater, an American biochemist and expert in trace elements, wrote a book on the subject called *Selenium as Food and Medicine* (Keats, 1980) and the British Arthritic Association carried out a clinical trial using selenium on some of their most disabled victims. At about the same time *Here's Health* magazine in Britain started to tell its readers about selenium and as a result knowledge was slowly amassed which pointed to the place that selenium was to hold as a health supplement of real value.

A back-track through history

In many ways the slow spread of knowledge about selenium reminds me of the vitamin C story. Way back in 1600 Sir James Lancaster, the British merchant and sea captain who took part in the defeat of the Spanish Armada and later commanded the first fleet of the East India Company, found he could keep his ships free of the devastating killer disease of scurvy simply by giving his crews the juice of lemons to drink on long journeys. Strangely this knowledge was not very well publicized and it fell to a naval doctor called James Lind to 'rediscover' that oranges and lemons prevented and cured the disease some years later. Later still Captain Cook showed that, provided he provisioned his boats with fresh fruits and vegetables from the islands he visited, his crews kept reasonably free from scurvy.

It is also odd that real scientific understanding of the vital part that vitamin C played in the prevention of scurvy was then 'forgotten' once again in the nineteenth century, and we had to wait until the first half of this century before the real facts of the matter became common medical knowledge.

Selenium 'discovered' at last — so let's not 'forget' it

Once again, lack of communication in the scientific journals together with scepticism about exactly how a trace element could influence health hampered widespread knowledge of selenium until quite recently. And, to a large extent, it was a sort of 'word of mouth' system that helped the early dissemination of knowledge of the subject (like the story of lemon juice and scurvy). *Here's Health* magazine was an early source of public knowledge on selenium and Alan Lewis's paperback on selenium *Selenium: The Facts About this Essential Mineral* (Thorsons, 1982) reinforced the message. In that book, now out of print, he published a selection of letters from readers who had been so impressed by selenium's action that they took the trouble to put pen to paper about it. They were mostly rheumatism sufferers, and there was a quality of sensible enthusiasm about what they wrote.

One such reader started his letter by voicing a general distrust of drugs, but found that after taking selenium for about three months his previously painful knees were a lot better and, although they still 'clicked', there was not the pain that there used to be. Another reader had been taking the often very effective non-steroidal anti-rheumatic drugs (some of which

What is selenium?

have had to be removed from the market recently due to dangerous side-effects). He found that he could switch to selenium and yet remain free from pain.

Another *Here's Health* reader had been battling for years with progressive arthritis of his hips. Scared of the much publicized drugs he had been prescribed he switched first to aspirin and then to selenium. After a brief flare-up of his symptoms, that lasted about a week, his pain started to settle. In eight weeks it had gone.

This 'slow action', together with the flare-up of symptoms phenomenon, is to a large extent a characteristic of trace element therapy. Another *Here's Health* reader had had arthritis for six years and took pain killers regularly. She could not lift anything around the house and although she lived only 50 yards from the shops she could no longer 'make it', and a neighbour had to do all the shopping for her. When she started on selenium she was initially disappointed by lack of any response. Encouraged to persevere, however, after about two months her pain started to ease. After four months of therapy she could walk again, and mobility returned to her shoulders. In her own words 'life was worthwhile again'.

This slow action phenomenon is entirely logical when you consider how the body reacts to all sorts of deficiencies. We know how, for instance, in the case of iron deficiency the body first of all mobilizes its stores of iron. Then, if the iron deficiency in the diet continues the tissue stores of iron start to fall and only eventually, when the body is seriously depleted in iron, do the symptoms of anaemia become manifest. If iron therapy is started, and provided absorption is adequate, symptoms gradually improve. But it may be months before the body's iron stores are replaced and the victim feels really well. And if absorption is poor (and it is often poor *because* of the anaemia) redressing the iron balance is a slow business.

We know little about the storage of selenium in humans, but in farm animals the highest concentrations of selenium are found in the liver and, surprisingly, in the kidneys too. It seems highly likely that these organs are also *our* selenium stores, although we await research findings on this score. It would seem likely, therefore, that in selenium deficiency these meagre stores (for we are still talking in trace element terms) are first of all diminished and then they become exhausted. Once this happens the ultimate tissue effects of selenium depletion start to produce the symptoms that are dealt with in detail later in this book.

But once selenium is taken it seems highly likely that, because of the previous depletion state, the very cells of the organ of absorption in the first few feet of our small intestine have themselves become ineffective and have great difficulty in absorbing the selenium we offer them. Exactly the same state of affairs occurs in iron deficiency where in some cases absorption is so poor that doctors have to give iron injections to boost the serum iron enough to coax the body back into something approaching normal as far as iron absorption is concerned.

Back at the factory

The introduction of selenium as a dietary supplement and the news about its efficacy and general helpfulness did not become obvious only at the editorial offices of health magazines. Understandably, it was also noted by the major manufacturers of selenium supplements and research into this trace element and its beneficial properties was stepped up.

For instance, an angina sufferer with the classic symptoms of angina pectoris (chest pain on exertion) found that after taking selenium supplementation for about a year her angina disappeared.

A woman who had severe menopausal symptoms, and who previously needed tranquillizers and sleeping tablets, found after six months' treatment that she could sleep on five nights out of six without sedatives. She also had much more energy and felt more relaxed without any drug therapy. She used the phrase 'good to be alive' in her spontaneous endorsement of selenium supplementation. Another elderly woman who had suffered for a number of years from chronic varicose leg ulcers found that, quite unexpectedly, her ulcers started to heal when she took selenium. After a year's therapy her chronic venous ulcers had totally healed and she was understandably enthusiastic about her cure.

Chronic pain is a depressing experience and the life of pain that has to be faced by many rheumatic sufferers is often very difficult to cope with. Selenium supplementation can also be helpful here. Although the majority of testimonials refer to improvements in the rheumatic condition itself, on long-term selenium supplementation, a minority mention that although the rheumatism itself was not demonstrably better the pain was easier to cope with. Selenium seemed to persuade many rheumatism sufferers to accept their pain almost as an 'old friend' and come to terms with it.

This *psychotrophic* effect of trace elements was first noticed by Dr Carl Pfeiffer, one of America's leading pioneers in the field of nutritional research, and he has investigated possible trace element abnormalities in schizophrenics in whom he demonstrates zinc deficiency, manganese deficiency (and copper excess). Dr Pfeiffer has held responsible professional positions in pharmacology and, although his work has not to date been reduplicated, it would seem likely that selenium deficiency has, as a result of neuro-enzyme derangement or upset, a link with diseases of the nervous system too.

CHAPTER 2
What's wrong with testimonials?

On the whole, and with a few notable exceptions, doctors are a pretty sensible lot. They go through a long and arduous training that often involves the sacrifice of many of the 'fun years' of youth to join a profession in which, although few are poor, very few reach a standard of living enjoyed by successful graduates in other professional and business fields.

If they are good doctors their training makes them careful, analytical and above all conservative in the management of their patients. As a result they are sensibly suspicious of medical 'breakthroughs', 'amazing new treatments' and most of the things that the popular press gets enthusiastic about. They are also very suspicious of testimonials. One of the reasons for this is that their training makes them first of all cognizant of the natural history of disease (in other words what happens to the patient if you give him nothing in the way of treatment) and secondly they are at pains to look for and take account of what is called the *placebo* response.

I will please

Placebo is Latin for *I will please* and in its original concept a placebo was looked upon as a treatment given to 'humour' the patient. Gradually, however, it has become obvious that the placebo response is something much more interesting than this because the 'humouring' factor is present and can be measured, even if drugs or treatment systems are being used that have no known therapeutic effect — or even effects that might be expected to make the patient's symptoms become rather worse!

Nowadays, when clinical trials of new drugs are being set up a 'blind' factor is built into the trial which hopefully takes into account this strange and 'inexplicable' placebo effect.

Write a testimonial: get into print

Another reason why doctors don't like testimonials is that when people take a 'new cure' on the advice of a friend, their next-door neighbour, an advertisement in a magazine, a television advertisement, or even as a result of reading a book they are sometimes encouraged to write a testimonial saying how fabulous their 'new cure' has been. The placebo response does not always get taken into consideration in such cases. Neither does the natural history of the disease. So a testimonial tends to lead to that very human frailty known as self-deception.

In the old days when the manufacturers of patent medicines were far more exploitative than they are today both advertisements for medicines and ointments and the actual bottles or tins that contained them were often plastered with testimonials. So much so that a well-known Canadian newspaper, the *Toronto Star*, once proclaimed 'if your brains won't get you into the papers try writing a patent medicine testimonial; maybe your kidneys will!' But the reason above all that makes doctors suspect the testimonial so much is that they fear that their patients are not sophisticated enough to appreciate the *post hoc propter hoc* (after this because of this) type of fallacy.

Years ago when I published *The Natural History of Quackery* (Michael Joseph, 1961) (shyly under the pseudonym of Eric Jameson, for it was in the days when doctors in practice were not supposed to write books in their own names) I explored the quack testimonial in some detail. In those 'bad old days' of the testimonial business the main principles of 'puffing' up claims to a cure were quite flagrant. One was to latch on to a popular figure, a sports hero for instance, and then claim that his prowess was due to this or that nostrum. For instance a medicine called Nuxated Iron which was promoted as a general tonic and cure-all 'signed up' the popular boxing hero Jack Dempsey, and for a while bottles of the tonic bore the legend that 'Nuxated Iron put him in the superb condition' that he could 'whip Jess Willard' (his opponent). Another good sell in the testimonial game was to obtain a personal endorsement from an eminent physician (the Pope's doctor actually signed a testimonial for Nuxated Iron). Retired generals, judges or film stars were much sought after and 'used' in this way!

I must admit that while collecting together examples of bogus testimonial activity I had a lot of fun and hopefully produced a few smiles from my readers whom I persuaded to look at testimonials in a new light of scepticism. In my enthusiasm for debunking patent medicine cures, however, I failed to see that every now and again the testimonial — the 'by word of mouth' endorsement — sometimes is the *only* way in which new medical knowledge becomes promulgated.

The amazing lady from Lynne

This is illustrated quite nicely I think in the story of Lydia Pinkham, otherwise known as the Lady from Lynne (Massachusetts). As a young medical student I used to sing at hospital 'bean feasts' the following ditty:

> And so we drink, we drink, we drink to Lydia Pink, Pink, Pink
> The saviour of the human race
> She invented a vegetable compound
> Efficacious in every case.

Usually this was accepted as something of an epitome of informed medical comment on patent medicines of every sort. Of course Mrs Pinkham's selling techniques, which made her eventually the first woman millionaire in the United States, was heavily promoted by testimonial-type advertising, and the American Medical Association attacked her roundly and persistently on this score.

Mrs Pinkham's famous compound was marketed mainly for what were euphemistically called, in those days, *female complaints*. In other words, it was for the various gynaecological ills that the female frame was heir to, including the symptoms of the menopause. Mrs Pinkham made many changes in the formulation of her famous 'vegetable compound' as the years went by, and pretty ruthlessly exploited the many testimonials she received from grateful patients. But we must remember that in her heyday medical treatment — and particularly gynaecological treatment — was pretty primitive and often quite horrendous, and so there was fair cause for so many American sufferers trying the famous medicine.

One reason for the success of Lydia Pinkham's famous compound was a very simple one — it worked! And this facet of 'do it yourself' health care is one that doctors, particularly, are keen to ignore or ridicule — or to dismiss as a 'placebo response'. But Lydia Pinkham's nostrum was found eventually to be based on a herbal remedy that was shown to have a measurable oestrogenic effect. It is lack of the naturally produced hormone called oestrogen which produces, at around the time of the change of life in women, the symptoms of the menopause that cause so much upset and distress. It is perhaps curious that plant products contain substances that profoundly affect animal tissues and human physiology. But there it is. (The major sources of the sex hormones used in the contraceptive pill are plants.) The reason that so many women wrote and told Mrs Pinkham about how the remedy had helped them was because the oestrogen substance in it *did* really help them. But it was quite a long time before the medical profession 'discovered' HRT (hormone replacement therapy) and started using oestrogens themselves! In the meanwhile Lydia Pinkham's remedy was widely criticized and made to look ridiculous.

Signs of (welcome) change

Changes in medical attitudes are often very slow, for doctoring is, as I said, a very conservative profession. As luck would have it I have been involved in the process of some of the important changes that have taken place in medical thinking with reference to health and nutrition over the last couple of decades or so, and almost by accident to some extent I have watched some interesting changes take place.

Scientists and pharmacologists who worked for the largest commercial producers of fish oils at Marfleet Refinery in Hull, were for a long time puzzled that their company received large numbers of letters (testimonials) from people who had found that the regular taking of cod liver oil improved their rheumatism. To my knowledge the company never used this mass of public endorsement to promote sales of cod liver oil as an anti-rheumatic treatment, but a best-selling book was published in the United States by Dan Alexander on the subject of the beneficial effects of cod liver oil for rheumatism. There is no doubt that word of mouth recommendations were responsible for its success.

Interest generated in Britain by *Here's Health* magazine was instrumental in the popularization of selenium as an anti-rheumatic and the manufacturers of a popular brand also found themselves at the receiving end of many testimonial letters. Before long a doctor wrote a testimonial about it that was published in the *Lancet*, a medical journal that is generally acknowledged to represent the opinions of the most influential medical scientists in the world.

The testimonial in question came from Dr Eldon W. Kienholz of the Department of Animal Sciences, Colorado State University. For three years he had suffered from ligament strain to his knee joint and this had been getting so bad that he had become unable to take part in his favourite recreation — mountain hiking. His doctors advised him to 'accept the situation' as there was no effective therapy available. Hearing by word of mouth that selenium relieved certain kinds of arthritis he began to take a selenium/vitamin E preparation. Six months later he was able to partake in an 11-mile hike that was much more strenuous in terms of hill climbing than the expedition he had found so very painful and disabling just one year previously.

Of course one enthusiastic and unsolicited testimonial means nothing even if it does get accepted by the *Lancet,* and a much more detailed examination of the part that selenium supplementation plays in the management of rheumatism is given in Chapter 6. All that we set out to explore in this preliminary chapter was the part that testimonials *can* play in the dissemination of medical treatment and why it is unrealistic to reject them out of hand as dubious contributions towards advances in medicine generally.

I find it fascinating that the vast majority of testimonials to selenium are devoid of the characteristics of the placebo response, the 'miracle cure' or the health craze. In no way is selenium some sort of instant cure for the ills of the world. Its action from the medical point of view is often slow to start and incidentally slow to fade once selenium is discontinued. It acts in other words not like a drug but like a nutrient — and nutrient deficiencies can present in many guises as will be demonstrated quite soon as we learn more about this extraordinary and interesting trace element.

CHAPTER 3
Trace elements and good health

Before we start to look in subsequent chapters at the sort of evidence that convinces even very sceptical doctors about the benefits of selenium, a few more basic facts about nutrients in general, and selenium in particular, must be examined, that is if we are going to realize just how important this whole subject is to our health and well-being.

When Walter de la Mare wrote his poem about 'whatever Miss T eats turns into Miss T' he was unconsciously, I am sure, giving us a paraphrase of the whole of Nutritional Science. Incredibly not too many people believe it! And yet when you think about it it *must* be true. The science of Nutrition merely breaks our constant and life-giving appetite for food into its constituent bits and pieces. Hopefully a closer look at some of these in more detail will help us to understand the vital facts of nutritional life a little better.

We know that the *proteins* in the animal and vegetable world that we eat are used mostly to build up our own tissues. We raid the world of plants and flowers for their energy stores, the (*carbohydrate*) sugars, starches and oils, to produce the *energy* we need, supplementing this with animal energy stores (fat and marine oil) too. It was tempting to believe that provided we got the protein, fat, carbohydrate balance right then health was ours for the asking, and then a little over 50 years ago the *vitamins* were 'invented'. It has indeed taken us quite a long while to learn about the less obvious world of nutrition which involves the part that even vitamins play in turning what we eat into 'Miss T'. As mentioned in a previous chapter we learnt (or relearnt) about most of the vitamins during the first half of the twentieth century. Now we really have to learn about the *minerals* that are also necessary to our health if we are to realize our natural good health potential.

Enter the RDA

Scientists, medical and otherwise, love technical terms that can be reduced to initials. And the Recommended Daily Allowance (RDA) is a prime example of this love affair in action. It came about as a result of laudable enough motives to enable people to check easily, at a glance, from a list, exactly how much of the various nutrients are advisable to guarantee good health.

This brought a certain warm inner feeling of confidence to the world of nutrition for a while. But not for long. The first sign of a fly in this otherwise soothing ointment came when it was realized that these RDAs apply only to *normal healthy individuals*. This looks fine at a first glance, but when you start to look *individuals* straight in the eye they become less of a comforting stereotype and more (yes you have guessed it) individual!

Any individual probably has food likes and dislikes and consequently eating habits will vary. He or she may or may not smoke and this can alter the way he or she uses food. He or she may or may not be over 40 or 50 or 60 or 70 and this influences the way food is absorbed. She may or may not take the contraceptive pill. Quite a lot of normal healthy individuals keep that way because they sensibly take, occasionally, prescribed medication. Others 'help themselves' with Over-The-Counter medication if they get a headache, a cold, run a fever, suffer a little indigestion or get period pains. From the point of view of everyday living this is fine but all these things can alter vitamin and mineral needs. So, if we are looking to RDAs for advice as to what's healthy in the way of mineral or vitamin intake, from the practical point of view your comforting RDA list becomes worthless.

Strangely perhaps the US Food and Nutrition Board of the National Academy of Science who produce what is probably the most influential list of RDAs that we have, assumes that there is a 2 to 3 per cent risk of deficiency of each and every nutrient occurring on the list if we slavishly adhere to RDAs. When one considers that there are possibly 30 essential nutrients needed to ensure good health it would seem reasonable to assume that to live by RDAs is to live quite dangerously at times.

The big absorption dilemma

As we gradually learn more about our nutritional requirements as *normal healthy individuals* it appears that the greatest and usually unknown factor is the very variable *individual absorption* of nutrients which occurs. This is often idiosyncratic. To start with, our knowledge on this score was based on animal experiments. For instance, evidence was found that in a group of 102 male guinea pigs there was a 20-fold range in their needs for vitamin C. A similar group of rats were shown to have a 3- to 10-fold variation in their requirements for vitamin A and folic acid, for instance.

As animal experiments like these progressed, it was established that genetic factors had a profound influence on the health needs of all laboratory animals. Sometimes it was possible to demonstrate that apparently arbitrary factors (like feather colour in chicks) were linked with quite considerable variations in the needs for vitamins to keep animals healthy and free from vitamin deficiency problems.

Always there are those who throw up their hands in anguish when we talk about evidence obtained from animal experiments and cry out that they do not believe in 'white mouse medicine'. There is something in what they say. Different species do live and die in very different ways. Human experimentation has, however, demonstrated that there are big differences in nutritional needs in the human animal too, and that these may well be genetic as well.

For example, one way in which it is possible to gauge when the human animal has become fully 'topped-up' with one vital nutrient, in this case vitamin C, is to measure how much vitamin C is excreted in the urine after a given dose of the vitamin is swallowed. If everybody absorbed vitamin C equally well and efficiently then the dose of vitamin C necessary for them to excrete a certain amount of the vitamin would be the same. However, in an experiment that involved nine normal adult women it was necessary for them to swallow doses that ranged from 42 to 154mg of vitamin C to excrete similar quantities of the vitamin in their urine — an interesting comment upon how variable is our capacity to absorb vitamin substances from our diet. Probably the same applies to minerals.

We now know that human needs for a whole range of nutrients vary substantially with all sorts of previously ignored factors. For instance, if we eat a lot of unsaturated fat (animal-derived fat) in our diet we need extra vitamin E to keep us fit and well. Disease, stress, trauma, infection and surgery all greatly affect our nutritional requirements. There is evidence that in some cases vitamin and mineral supplementation far in excess of RDAs speeds recovery of those who have undergone surgery, sustained fractures or suffered burns.

The twentieth-century dilemma

In many ways we in the western world are very well off nutritionally. We get enough protein to build and service our bodies. We certainly get enough carbohydrate to provide us with an abundant energy bank — so much so that many of us can't spend enough of the energy at our disposal and we get over-fat on stored energy as a result. As far as fat is concerned we are in a difficult position. We eat it seems too much animal fat to be good for us and not enough marine oil and so our bodies tend to get out of balance fat-wise and prone to many animal-fat-induced diseases (for example a tendency towards coronary heart disease).

But, as far as minerals and vitamins are concerned even the affluent western man and woman brimming with nutritional wealth in some ways is at risk from malnutrition in others. Because we derive over 60 per cent of our calories from purified sugars, animal fat, milled grains, and alcohol, and because we cook (sometimes more than once) most of the food we eat, we continually hover on the edge even of RDAs as far as minerals and vitamins are concerned and we have seen how unreliable RDAs are in protecting our health. In fact, if we ate all our food raw it would seem that Nature would give us four times our present RDAs of vitamins and minerals — an interesting comment on the sophistication of eating practices spelling ruination of really healthy eating.

Before leaving this interesting if somewhat hair-raising comment on everyday life and living, it is necessary to stress that all these factors that head us along the road towards modern malnutrition in the western world are accentuated in the elderly who really need a special range of RDAs all of their own to be on the safe side as far as health and longevity are concerned. To date nobody has concocted one. It could make uncomfortable reading!

Back to selenium

Everything we have been saying with reference to nutrition and RDAs in general applies especially to selenium, and an RDA for selenium has been suggested to be in the 50 to 200 microgram range (in the ninth edition of the US National Academy of Science List in 1980). This is roughly in tune with a (British) Ministry of Agriculture Fisheries and Food report that suggested an ideal daily intake of between 80 and 200 micrograms. Bearing in mind all the potential problems of RDAs that we have already dealt with, how does this look with reference to how we are being catered for as far as selenium is concerned? In other words are we eating enough selenium to turn us into fit and healthy 'Miss Ts'? From the available evidence it seems highly likely that we are not.

If we consult the following list of foodstuffs, produced to show exactly how we can eat our way into adequate selenium nutrition, it would seem at first glance that most of us should be getting enough. But this simply demonstrates how erroneous first impressions can be.

Sources of selenium
(Shortlist of US values)

Micrograms (mcg) per 100g edible portion (100g = 3½ oz)			
Butter	146	Eggs	21
Smoked herring	141	Orange juice	19
Smelt	123	Gelatin	19
Wheatgerm	111	Beer	19
Brazil nuts	103	Beef liver	18
Apple cider vinegar	89	Lamb chop	18
Scallops	77	Egg yolk	18
Barley	66	Mushrooms	12
Wholewheat bread	66	Chicken	12
Lobster	65	Swiss cheese	10
Bran	63	Cottage cheese	5
Shrimp	59	Wine	5
Red swiss chard	57	Radishes	4
Oats	56	Grape juice	4
Clams	55	Pecans	3
Crab	51	Hazelnuts	2
Oysters	49	Almonds	2
Milk	48	Green beans	2
Cod	43	Kidney beans	2
Brown rice	39	Onion	2
Topside steak	34	Carrots	2
Lamb	30	Cabbage	2
Turnips	27	Orange	1
Garlic	25		

Butter looks good as a source of selenium, but in the interests of health it is not a good idea to eat more than about ½ oz of butter per day.

Other rich selenium sources are fish, but here we come up against a difficult absorption problem because the selenium in fish tends to occur in conjugation with mercury which inhibits the body's absorption and so the real biological yield to our tissues is liable to be only a fraction of what is indicated in the table. When we consider milk, bread and meat as likely sources of selenium we must consider exactly how we eat these foods in order to get our RDA of 50 to 200 micrograms. Because selenium and selenium-containing compounds are very easily vaporized, anything we do in the way of cooking these selenium-rich basics diminishes their selenium content greatly. Bread is often eaten as toast, milk gets boiled or par-boiled in most milk drinks. Very few of us eat our meat raw. And, of course, the same applies to most of the other foods on our selenium shopping list.

Before leaving this brief exercise in shopping for selenium, a word about a curious member of the list we have quoted — apple cider vinegar. This does have a relatively high selenium content as you can see, but to get your RDA of selenium you would have to swallow quite a lot of the stuff. I mention this because some years ago a doctor from Vermont in the United States wrote a best-selling book called *Folk Medicine** in which he sung the praises loud and strong of apple cider vinegar and persuaded many of his readers that wherever this substance was a regular part of their diet so was health, fitness and longevity. Nobody, least of all Dr Jarvis, who put forward this 'cure', really knew just how something that appeared to be so innocuous therapeutically as apple cider vinegar could be a health bonus. Perhaps now at long last we know that there was something turning into the 'Miss T' of all those patients of Dr Jarvis that was doing them good — and that substance was selenium.

---

* D. C. Jarvis, *Folk Medicine*, (Pan, 1971).

CHAPTER 4
Medical geography and selenium

Richard Passwater, writing his definitive book on selenium*, drew some quite startling conclusions as a result of using what was then a little-known tool of medical investigation, called 'medical geography'. He started by linking low soil selenium levels to the disease that most of us dread above all others — cancer. We shall return to that subject later in this book. It is worthwhile for us to examine the very modern if neglected subject of medical geography in a little detail now because it sheds new light on some of the more puzzling problems of health and disease on a world-wide basis and in a way that is very relevant to our subject.

Incredibly, perhaps, there is only one well-established department of medical geography in the whole world that specializes in this emerging discipline. It is at the University of Washington in Seattle, and in a recent article (1984) in the *Journal of the American Medical Association* one of the department's key researchers Dr Johnathan D. Mayer explained how looking at the world through the medical geographer's eyes explains medical mysteries that have puzzled doctors for many years.

New developments in medical geography with health in mind

Several new geographic techniques have been developed with this aim in view. One of these involves a special analysis of diseases that goes far beyond the excellent early disease 'dot' maps that Richard Passwater used to introduce his readers to the fascinating world of 'this is where you live, so this is the sort of illness you are liable to suffer from' credo. Nowadays with computerized statistics using graphics software we can produce computer-designed maps that are indistinguishable from the old

---

* Richard Passwater, *Selenium as Food and Medicine*, (Keats, 1980).

laboriously constructed 'dot' maps very quickly, efficiently and cheaply. These can be up-graded at the touch of a button when fresh information comes to hand.

Another fascinating aspect of this new medical discipline is known as 'disease ecology'. Disease ecology is concerned with the myriad interactions that can occur between environment, culture and sickness. We shall see how acid rain and soil selenium are related in this 'ecological' concept a little later.

The fact that culture, as well as how people live and work, can influence disease is one of the most under-researched areas of medicine only now being fully appreciated. For instance, we know that in Britain the further you drift down the social scale the more likely you are to have a coronary thrombosis. But nobody has the slightest idea precisely why this should be!

Medical geography is, however, starting to solve some of these problems elsewhere in the world and Dr Jacques May, who is medical geographer at the American Geographical Society in New York City, has carried out some remarkable work particularly relevant to the geography of malnutrition.

Dr May has pointed out that whenever disease occurs there is a coming together in time and space of two factors. One is a disease *stimulus* which comes from the environment, the other is the *response* of the potential victim to that stimulus. He is also at pains to point out that disease 'challenges' vary with the cultural and social climate.

Examples make this concept of the ecology of disease easier to understand.

We know for instance that contact with the tsetse fly causes the disease we call trypanosomiasis, or sleeping sickness. But although the tsetse fly is found widely in Africa it is only in parts of sub-Sahara Africa that trypanosomiasis is a real health problem. This is because the landscape characteristics (non-medical geography) of certain sub-Sahara regions bring relatively large numbers of people in contact with a *microenvironment* that is particularly hospitable to tsetse flies. An even more obvious cultural, one might almost say commercial, factor operating in disease incidence occured in Trinidad where (inexplicably) labourers in the cocoa plantations suddenly started to develop malaria. Now, we know that malaria is caused by human contact with the anopheline mosquito — a regular resident of the Trinidad area. Why therefore the sudden epidemic in cocoa workers? Well, payment in the cocoa fields

Medical geography and selenium

became so poor that most workers got other jobs to occupy themselves during the day and worked in the cocoa plantations (you might honestly say 'moonlighted' in this context) only in the early evenings. Now it is in the early evenings that the malarial mosquitoes like to feed and so the cocoa workers developed malaria in large numbers. A similar 'epidemic' of malaria occurred in Malaysia some years ago when extensive wood clearance took place for extension of the rubber plantations. This removed dense light-filtering arboreal canopies and allowed sunlight to flood into areas that had previously been dark and lightless. This allowed pools of warm water to occur in the newly cultivated areas and warm pools of water are exactly what mosquitoes like to breed in, and so an epidemic of malaria developed.

One new and important lesson that medical geography has to teach us is obvious when we look at the relationship of selenium deficiency in our soil to the incidence of acid rain.

Selenium starts in the soil

Leaving aside fish-derived selenium, before selenium can get into us it has first of all to get into the cereals that we eat, or the cereals that the animals that become meat to us eat, that is unless we add to our diet (as an increasing number of people do) a selenium supplement. There is no other way that selenium can get 'into Miss T'. Now, whenever maps of soil selenium content are made there is evidence of increasing selenium depletion occurring. This happens particularly wherever there is extensive prairie-type farming, especially when this is supported by the heavy use of artificial fertilizers. But there is also evidence of very low soil selenium in another type of area, and this is particularly pertinent to Britain and certain parts of northern Europe: the areas affected by acid rain.

Dead fish now — dead people next?

Acid rain has become a big political issue in Europe and the Green (ecology) party in Germany particularly has started to wield some power in government on the issue of acid rain. Not everybody, by a long chalk, understands exactly what acid rain is, although they know that all over Europe it is leading to dead forests. Woodlands play a particularly important part in the folklore of continental Europe as well as in its economy. Unfortunately we in Britain are partially culpable; we add to the European acid rain problem as our power station and industrial pollution often seems to get wafted across the North Sea into the skies of Europe.

It appears that few of us in this country worry too much about dead trees. But we are more concerned about dead fish, or rather the total absence of fish in lochs and lakes where once they were abundant — as a result of acid rain. The same applies on the other side of the Atlantic Ocean.

It has been calculated that in the United States, where an increasing number of citizens are also getting worried about the effects of acid rain, around 50 million metric tonnes of sulphur and nitrogen oxides are being released into the skies every year as a result of the combustion of fossil fuels — in other words coal and oil (including petrol) — and that, through a series of complex chemical reactions going on in the clouds above us, these substances are converted into acids that produce the devastating impact on our environment.

In Britain, somehow, our ecologists are not producing enough hard information on this score to publicize the facts effectively. But elsewhere in the world ecology is hitting the politicians hard and exactly where it hurts them — in the ballot box! The citizens of New York State have traditionally enjoyed fishing on the picturesque lakes of the Adirondack mountains until recently. Now more than ninety of the best lakes are fishless due to acid rain, and legislation is being forced through to combat this — but of course very slowly!

It has only recently been realized that acid rain has an effect on soil selenium and so is contributing to all the diseases of selenium depletion we will be examining in later chapters. In a nutshell the increasing use of fossil fuel, and especially coal burning in UK power stations, diminishes the amount of selenium that plants can absorb from the soil. This is reflected in turn in a lowered selenium content in cereals and in everyone who lives either directly or indirectly on those cereals. Dr Douglas Frost writing in *Annual Reviews of Pharmacology* has demonstrated that there has been a progressive decline in soil selenium on a year-by-year basis in the USA, and doubtless the same is true in Europe. Acid rain is one of the reasons for this. It can be counteracted by more efficient emission control, but this adds slightly to the costs of electricity. The costs ultimately to the human frame are difficult to over-estimate.

——Medical geography and food and drink——

Some of the most baffling of medical problems have been solved by the application of a little medical geography. The disease we know as gout is basically a disorder of uric acid metabolism, and by avoiding foods high in uric acid and by taking medicines that help the body to rid itself of excess uric acid most sufferers can these days keep themselves free of this nasty disease. Gout was, of course, known to the Romans who knew nothing of modern biochemistry. They did know, however, that the drinking of certain alcoholic products tended to precipitate an attack of gout and that certain wines were particularly prone to do this. This form of gout was a total mystery for years. A little knowledge of medical geography would have solved the mystery a long while ago, however. The wine that gave the gout was wine that was fermented using soft water and lead-lined fermentation or storage tanks. This allowed the wine to contain more than a little lead as a trace element. This lead disturbed the body's ability to deal with uric acid which subsequently became deposited in joints and other tissues giving the symptoms of gout.

——Selenium in food——

An appraisal of modern medical geography can give us an idea as to where we might expect to find enough selenium to keep us fit and well, or where the intake of selenium is liable to be deficient. As mentioned previously the RDA (recommended daily allowance) of selenium is thought to be within the range of 50 to 200 micrograms per day. The National Academy of Science in the USA puts it lower at between 20 and 60 micrograms per day. But selenium intake in food varies throughout the world, as medical geography shows, from reasonably high levels to those which contain only half as much selenium deemed necessary to provide optimum protection against cancer for instance.

Research that originated from the Ministry of Agriculture in England puts the average British intake at 60 micrograms per day. Half of this comes from cereals and cereal products and the rest from meat and fish. Other countries have widely different selenium intakes with ranges that give real cause for anxiety. For example New Zealand has a low intake of about 25 micrograms per day and Sweden's ranges from between 23 and 210 micrograms per day.

When isolated groups of people are looked at with reference to their selenium intake alone (and this does not take into consideration known variations in selenium absorption) quite worrying statistics emerge. When Dr Douglas Frost, who did an analytical survey on a large series of (institutional) meals, subjecting them to selenium analysis by sophisticated photofluorometric studies he detected no selenium at all in most of them!

CHAPTER 5
Selenium and life extension

When Alan Lewis leaped onto his transcultural 'bike' a few years ago in search of knowledge of life extension, he came up with some extraordinary stories of longevity (*Selenium: The Facts About This Essential Mineral,* Thorsons, 1982). To start with he introduced us to Leon Ojeda and Miguel Corpio. I must admit that I had never heard of them, but that was understandable for they both lived in remote areas in South America where they had survived to incredible ages. Of course, when people are born, live and die in places of the world where population statistics are as rare as bacon sandwiches at a bar mitzvah, it is sensible always to take tales of longevity with more than an average-sized pinch of salt! In the case of Leon and Miguel it seems to have been pretty carefully checked out that they lived for a very long time, but whether they were really 130 and 123 we will never know.

Both of these men were residents of the Andes, however, and the area does enjoy a reputation for substantial numbers of ultra senior citizens, as does the Vilcabamba Valley in Ecuador, the Southern Caucasus in the Soviet Union, and the Unza section of Pakistan.

Dr David Davies, a physician from the Gerontology Department at University College London, has given a deal of credence to many of the claims that have hailed from Ecuador on this scene, for he has related baptismal certificates, vouched for by priests, to at least four people who died 150 years later! When the diets of these people were examined by Dr Davies they were seen to be austere, monotonous and vegetarian. But they had another characteristic — all the food was eaten raw or nearly raw. Now, of course, there are nutritional advantages and disadvantages to a diet of raw food that we have not the space to go into very much at the moment. One advantage is, however, that food eaten raw will contain *all* the selenium that nature endows it with. None disappears in the cooking. And the geography of this area of Ecuador suggests that they may well enjoy a high selenium soil there too.

Alan Lewis also delved usefully into the diet of the famous centenarians of Russia, living as they do mostly in the mountains on the Russo-Iranian border. Here a multinational team of Russian, French and American scientists busied themselves in one village of 1,200 inhabitants where there were 71 men and 110 women between the ages of 81 and 90. Nineteen were over 90 and several were centenarians. Basically these folk were Abkasian nomads who lived mostly on fruit, beans and root vegetables well-flavoured with garlic which is, incidentally, selenium-rich. Sugar is never eaten and meat eating is rare. Nutritionally this would amount to a low-fat high-fibre diet and again one rich in natural minerals, especially selenium.

The Hunzas of Pakistan, who also claim more than a fair share of aged and very active citizens among their numbers, also eat a largely vegetable diet rich in pulses and low in meat.

Geography rather than 'vegetable-ography' the clue

It is always sensible, when looking at strange tales of health and longevity coming from far-away places and strange-sounding diets, continually to be on the *qui vive* for fallacy and to be sure exactly *what* you are looking at. Dr Roland Phillips who compared the life and death statistics of two religious groups did just that. His conclusions were really very interesting. There are doctrinal similarities between the Seventh Day Adventists and the Mormons. They both enjoy a similar lifestyle in many ways, prohibiting alcohol and smoking, for instance. But Seventh Day Adventists are, generally speaking, vegetarians as opposed to the Mormons who eat meat. When Dr Phillips presented his research on these two communities at a special symposium on cancer and nutrition it was tempting to link meat-eating to cancer as the Seventh Day Adventists developed cancer less frequently than did the Mormons.

But Dr Phillips did not stop his researches at this point. He also showed that among the Mormons there were interesting variations in the cancer rate geographically. One group of theoretically cancer-prone meat-eating Mormons had in fact a very low cancer rate — they were the Mormons who lived around Utah. Medical geography has discovered that this Utah area has a very high level of selenium in the soil. This it could be reasonable to assume was acting as a cancer preventative. More about this in Chapter 8.

Geography and health in Britain

Unfortunately medical geography is virtually in its infancy in the United Kingdom although it has been found that in the country around Upper Sheringham in East Anglia there are two to three times as many people over the age of 75 than in the country as a whole.

If we compare these Norfolk 'long-livers' with those that we have been examining rather superficially in very far away places, there are several similarities, the most striking of which is lack of industrialization and a habit of eating a lot of home-grown vegetable produce. But, of course, the main dramatic similarity is that by some sort of geographical accident they also enjoy living on a high soil selenium area and so get a lot of selenium in their locally grown food.

The vital link and science

Is it possible to link scientifically a tendency to slow down the rate of ageing and selenium intake? Until comparatively recently your hard-headed scientist would carefully wrap himself around with his long white coat and say 'definitely not'. Today such rejection is much less prevalent. But before we look at the problem in a little more detail it is necessary to try to work out a scientific definition of what we mean by ageing so that, once again, we know *exactly* what we are talking about.

First of all there are two types of ageing and it is convenient to look at ageing under the headings of (i) random and (ii) planned ageing. Random ageing is what 'happens' to us you might say. And this is to some extent under our control. The easiest type of random ageing is seen in what happens if we expose our skin to high doses of sunshine for longer than is good for us. You can see this sort of random ageing in action if you look at the faces of middle-aged women-folk in Australia and California where the cult of sun worship tends to reign supreme. Constant over-exposure to ultra-violet light destroys the skin's subcutaneous elastic tissue and the skin looks old much too soon for its chronological status. X-rays do the same sort of thing, and so do certain chemicals and pharmaceuticals (notably hydrocortisone ointments).

Another type of random ageing reaction occurs as a result of the reaction on our body of agents known as *free radicals*. I will explain these in more detail shortly for we can do something about this problem.

Planned ageing is really Nature's seemingly unkind obsolescence system in action. It is unkind to us (as individuals) but is built into the system of natural biology to make sure that the species survives. If you want to have a quick and ready example of planned ageing in action you cannot do better than to look at the menopause which occurs right on time in a large majority of women around the age of 50.

There is a certain amount of evidence that we can make certain alterations even in planned ageing and Durk Pearson and Sandy Shaw argued eloquently on this score in their fascinating book on life extension.*

Random ageing controlled

Some of this control is really a matter of self-control and slowly realizing that if you want to see a woman with a nice young-looking face when she's sixty-plus she cannot do better than go to a nunnery and observe the effect of living under the protection of a permanent sunshade for most of her life!

Other ways of slowing down random ageing involve avoiding the ill-effects of those free radicals mentioned earlier. To understand more about this important process it is necessary to concentrate for a little while on one of the basic elements of all living matter — and a lot of dead matter too. It is the element oxygen. Of course we need masses of oxygen to breathe to keep us alive. We use it to produce the energy we need to keep our bodies going, and there is every possible reason for considering oxygen one of the staffs of life as far as most of the animal world is concerned.

Now mostly when we use oxygen in our body, as the main currency of biologic energy, we convert it into water and the simple chemical equation that states: O_2 (oxygen) plus H_2 (hydrogen) $= H_2O$ plus energy is basic to our existence. But due to all sorts of complex biological reasons not *all* the oxygen in the air we breathe finishes up as water. Some of it turns into hydrogen peroxide (yes, the stuff 'peroxide blondes' used to bleach their hair with) and in this process oxygen produces some of those *free radicals* we mentioned earlier.

These oxygen-derived free radicals can attack all sorts of body tissues, particularly lipid membranes and DNA (the basic 'stuff' of cell reduplication) and certain other vital cell proteins too.

Of course, Nature would not have devised free radicals for nothing. And, of course, free radicals do good as well as bad. The phagocytes that scavenge up all sorts of unwelcome intruders into our body mobilize

---

* Durk Pearson and Sandy Shaw, *Life Extension*, (Warner Books, 1981).

free radicals and convert them into biological 'Exocet missiles' that seek out invading bacteria and kill them. However, there is increasing awareness, as Dr J. F. Nunn of the Clinical Research Centre at Harrow, Middlesex, pointed out in the *British Journal of Clinical Practice* recently, that oxygen-derived free radicals are the final common pathway that is walked in the production of much tissue damage. Free radicals make a contribution to ageing too.

Our bodies are in many ways a bit like fighting ships blasting off bacteria-seeking free radicals, but at the same time forced to keep a 'decoy helicopter' hovering around to deflect any free radicals from turning in on themselves. Instead of helicopters we produce enzymes. These enzymes can be obligingly 'initialized' in many instances. For example, there is SOD (which saves us having to remember how to spell superoxide dismutase). Another one similarly becomes CAT (the tissue enzyme catalase). In addition the body has the ability to scavenge free radicals by a system based on another enzyme called GLUP, or glutathione peroxidase if you wish to be precise. Other scavenger systems and antioxidants also include Vitamin C, Vitamin E and — as it happens — selenium.

The more we look into the chemical identity of enzyme systems in our bodies the more we learn about the way our bodies work. This is particularly well illustrated with reference to GLUP. Although selenium is not too widely distributed throughout the body, glutathione peroxidase, that anti-ageing scavenger of dangerous free radicals, contains four atoms of selenium and cannot be produced in the body unless enough selenium is freely available.

Occasionally genetic defects occur in children which result in someone missing out on this or that enzyme system. One such condition is the rare disease of progeria which is characterized by extremely rapid pathological ageing in which victims die at around puberty showing many of the classical signs of old age.

Those of us who have become increasingly convinced that selenium is an enormously important micronutrient were heartened to read in the *Lancet* recently that two reports in the world's scientific literature had laid to rest any doubts about the importance of selenium in human metabolism. The reports referred to came from the People's Republic of China where selenium had solved a baffling problem of an epidemic of heart disease and also from New Zealand where selenium had cured a particularly nasty form of muscle weakness in patients on intravenous feeding. In both of these instances the indigenous population had a low intake of selenium and really their cure involved the solution of a problem of medical geography. At last we seem to be seeing how selenium can partially 'stop the clock' of ageing and it looks as though in doing this its powerful role as an antioxidant is being demonstrated.

Closely associated with the action of oxidants is the phenomenon of *cross linking*. What is it that leather, stale bread, superannuated windscreen wipers, 'elderly' plastic-covered garden furniture, the skin on the back of your hand and your forehead and perhaps even the tissues of your arteries have in common? The answer is the same ageing process called *cross linking*. Basically it is a biochemical process in which proteins lose their flexibility. Subsequently the biological blueprints that are characterized in DNA and RNA become blurred, giving faulty instructions to our cells, particularly our cell proteins.

It is thought that cross-linking damage to DNA is a principal cause of ageing. As we grow older the whole body becomes stiffer, less 'elastic', less resilient and less agile. In the same way as your windscreen wiper rubber no longer conforms to the complicated and subtle curve of your car windscreen, and starts to screech as it smudges rather than wipes, our tissues at a molecular level fall foul of cross linking too.

One way to get a rough and ready guide as to where you are at the present relative to cross linking in your body is to place your hand palm down on a table and lift a 'pinch' of the skin on the back of your hand and hold it there for five seconds. In a young person on release the pinch obliterates itself in seconds. In older folk the ridge of skin distortion takes much longer to disappear and just how much longer demonstrates just how far cross linking has aged your body. This little experiment would be just a depressing reminder of our ultimate morbidity and mortality if it were not for just one thing. We do have at our disposal today antioxidants like selenium, Vitamin C and Vitamin E that delay the process of cross linking. And so selenium supplementation becomes an important process of looking, feeling and staying younger than your years.

CHAPTER 6
Beating arthritis with selenium

Arthritis and rheumatism are pretty vague terms, although sufferers know exactly what they mean in the way of pain and disability. But often the whole subject is blurred even in a doctor's consulting room, and patients will say almost apologetically: 'I think it's only a touch of rheumatism doctor,' as they rub their knee or elbow, or: 'It's not arthritis, is it doctor?' with fear in their hearts. This being so, a few definitions are worthwhile, once again, to be sure that we know *exactly* what we are talking about.

The term rheumatism was coined in the seventeenth century by doctors who knew precious little about medical science. They fancied that rhematic disease was caused by 'noxious vapours'. Now vapours do spread about, and rheumatism tends unfortunately to spread about the body too. The Greek root *rhe-* means 'to flow' and so we must excuse our medical ancestors for thinking they had hit on a pretty apt term to describe the agony of rheumatism.

A little later on in history as doctors learned more about disease they noticed how often inflammation of the tissues was involved when people got ill. To imply that inflammation was causing a medical problem they started putting *itis* after words. And so we got appendicitis, sinusitis, cholecystitis and of course arthritis. Now there are some pretty rare inflammatory arthritises, like septic arthritis and gout. But a great deal of all arthritis has nothing to do with inflammation at all and this is the case in the commonest form of arthritis, to whit — osteoarthritis.

The arthritis that isn't really an 'itis'

Osteoarthritis is a slowly progressive degeneration usually of one or two of the larger joints of the body, especially the hips and knees. It is so common in older people that it is often dismissed as a 'fair wear and tear' disease. A characteristic of the disease is the formation of spurs or lumps around the margins of the joints. Whatever initiates a joint becoming osteoarthritic (and nobody really knows why it happens) the trouble starts in the cartilage between the bones that make up the joint. This cartilage is usually a smooth and glistening tissue, but when osteoarthritis begins it becomes swollen and starts to degenerate. Cracks appear like they do on an ageing patch of concrete. This cracked cartilage then gets worn away and instead of a smooth gliding surface between the bones a rough and often unstable joint develops. The body reacts to this by laying down new bone around the edge of the joint in an attempt to make the joint more stable. Rarely does this help in any way.

During the early stages of osteoarthritis there are few symptoms and in fact an x-ray can show really advanced degrees of osteoarthritis and yet the patient happily remains symptom-free! This is because the cartilage and bone inside the joint have few pain receptors. Then a change starts to take place signalled usually by stiffness in the mornings, or after sitting for a long period say in a car or in the theatre or a restaurant. Usually these symptoms are worse in cold damp weather. Soon now pain sets in. This is because the 'new bone' that the body has been laying down has begun to press on sensitive tissues such as the synovial membrane (which secretes the joint's own lubricating fluid), the joint capsule or its ligaments. Eventually muscles become strained and the whole unpleasant business of an osteoarthritic joint has arrived.

Routine management

This is pretty stereotyped and is often quite effective. If the patient is overweight he or she is usually advised to go on a 1,400-calorie-per-day diet of a high-protein high-fibre type.* This will gradually allow the weight to fall even if the victim has been rendered relatively immobile by his or her disease. Physiotherapy based around the use of heat and carefully graduated exercises is helpful too. Because hospital physiotherapy departments are so over-crowded, 'home-physio' is often advised. Hot baths are excellent and so are hot showers and the intelligent use of electric blankets. Drug therapy is often helpful and both aspirin and the newer types of anti-rheumatic remedies (the non-steroidal anti-inflammatory drugs, often shortened to NSAIDs) are prescribed. Unfortunately there is a relatively high level of side-effects associated with the use of these drugs.

* Such diets are described in my book *The Complete Book of Slimming and Diets*, published by Piatkus Books.

The other big and unpleasant form of rheumatism is called rheumatoid arthritis. It affects younger age groups and is another common cause of pain and disability striking down some 150,000 folk per year in the UK alone.

Rheumatism proper

For many people rheumatism *is* rheumatoid arthritis, and this disease is quite different from osteoarthritis in all sorts of ways. It is not a disease of one or two joints but a generalized condition involving both multiple joints and many other organs or tissues throughout the body as well. Often it starts with mild aching or stiffness, more noticeable in the mornings. But as well as this patients usually complain of being tired and run down.

During the course of the disease 'rheumatic' joints may 'flare up'. They then become tender and swollen and in contrast to the case of osteoarthritis the joints most commonly involved are the smaller and more remote joints — the fingers, the wrists or the joints of the foot. Sometimes the disease will settle down in (shall we say) the fingers, only to reappear in the elbow or shoulder. The main part of the joint that seems to be 'suffering' is the synovial membrane or joint lining. This gets engorged and swollen so much that instead of being an entirely inconspicuous structure it becomes so enlarged and tender that it can be felt to bulge around the joint. In time this abnormal synovial membrane whose normal function is to lubricate and generally nourish the joint seems to develop a destructive nature and tends to 'eat away' the smooth joint cartilage. When this happens abnormal amounts of fluid collect in the joints increasing the local swelling.

The disease of rheumatoid arthritis is not limited to joints, however. It can 'invade' tendons and their sheaths restricting the movement of fingers. Sometimes tendons can even break and 'dropped fingers' become evident. Rheumatoid disease sometimes moves into the skin causing lumps or 'nodules'. Rarely, other organs of the body are affected as well.

What causes rheumatism?

This is really the $64,000 question! Despite intensive reseach throughout the world we know about as much of real value about this disease as we do about the common cold. We do know, however, some factors that are associated with an outpouring of rheumatic symptoms. Physical or mental stress may be involved. It may occur after childbirth or at the change of life. Strangely, during pregnancy a woman's rheumatism may spontaneously clear up, suggesting that hormones play an important part in the disease.

The most popular modern concept of rheumatism is that it is an autoimmune disease. What does this mean? Well, when the body is attacked by bacteria or viruses there is a swift response by our immune system to repel the potential invader (see also Chapter 10). If this did not happen we would die. Part of this reaction is made by specialized blood cells called lymphocytes. When these lymphocytes come into contact with the invading threat (called an antigen) they become transformed into what are called plasma cells. These produce antibodies which disable the invaders which can then be engulfed by another set of specialized blood cells called the phagocytes. In rheumatoid arthritis this immune reaction seems to become upset and disorganized.

One theory as to how this comes about is as follows. First of all, some sort of invading threat (with its *antigenic* component) somehow or other enters the body. (Maybe it is already in the body but lying dormant.) This combines in the usual way with lymphocytes to produce plasma cells which form antibodies. These antibodies now link with the antigen but for some unknown reason phagocytes go on to attack a joint's synovial membrane which develops the typical changes of rheumatoid arthritis.

Rheumatism management

After diagnosis and assessment a rheumatologist usually plans a therapeutic package for his patient which includes pain-killing drugs, anti-inflammatory drugs and specific anti-rheumatic remedies such as gold, steroids, penicillamine and anti-malarials. Always treatment has to be tailor-made to fit the patient. Side-effects are anticipated and as far as possible avoided. Alongside drug treatment, physical treatment with splints and standard physiotherapy are planned over a longish time scale.

Rheumatologist Dr U. Tarp and his colleagues, carrying out research at the Rheumatism Research Unit at Aahus in Denmark last year, have demonstrated that serum selenium levels in a group of 87 patients suffering from severe rheumatoid arthritis were significantly lower than in normal subjects. Patients with milder degrees of rheumatism showed a less reduced selenium level. Dr Ulrik Tarp, like all good rheumatologists, is cautious in the conclusions he draws from this new knowledge, but suggests that low activity of the selenium-dependent enzyme, glutathione peroxidase may be related to high levels of peroxidation products in rheumatoid arthritis. He also feels that patients with low selenium levels in their blood may develop more severe disease and cautiously endorses selenium supplementation in rheumatoid arthritis.

——A more natural management of arthritis——

Understandably rheumatism sufferers are not always too happy with their conventional treatments and the whole history of rheumatism management is peppered with 'alternative medicine' claims for this or that particular fringe or holistic therapy in such a nasty painful and disabling disease. Regrettably all too often what has looked like an exciting therapeutic 'breakthrough' for one particular new therapeutic approach to the condition of rheumatism, has been followed by disappointments on a long-term basis.

The possibility that selenium might be helpful in the long-term management of rheumatism seems to have sprung from veterinary medicine. Dr Richard Passwater, who has been a world-wide selenium watcher for over a decade, reported that as long ago as 1976 veterinarians in the United States were alleviating arthritic pain or swelling in animals with a product containing selenium and vitamin E. He was also one of the first scientists to suggest that the free radicals that we met in the last chapter were involved somehow in the rheumatic process as well.

Dr Passwater suggests that the superoxide dismutase (SOD) enzyme system holds the key to the anti-inflammatory free radical quenching that helps to settle arthritis down. In this view he is supported by Dr James L. Goddard, a former US Assistant Surgeon General. SOD is present in our tissues in relatively high quantities and, in fact, it is the fifth most abundant protein substance in our bodies after collagen, albumin, globulin and haemoglobin. In the United States, vets in charge of expensive racehorse stables frequently use selenium to mobilize SOD when their priceless thoroughbreds develop potentially disabling rheumatic symptoms.

This theory that free radicals are involved in the rheumatic process has gained support recently on several fronts. One conventional antirheumatic treatment already mentioned (penicillamine) seems to work because it chelates ('mops-up') certain metallic ions in the body that are capable of stimulating free radical production. High doses of antioxidants are capable of helping in rheumatoid disease. Pearson and Shaw mention, in their book on life extension, a rheumatic sufferer who could control his acute rheumatic disease by taking vitamin E but only in large doses (of 10,000–20,000 international units per day) thereby risking muscle weakness and proneness to fatigue, palpitation and increase in blood pressure due to over-dosage of vitamin E.

The Arthritic Association rheumatism trial (and why it worked)

The Arthritic Association is a patients' self-help group that keeps an open mind about new ways and treatments that may help sufferers from rheumatism in general. Its President, Charles Ware, is himself an arthritis sufferer who has lived with an arthritic hip for very nearly 50 years. By chance he decided to take a course of selenium in an organic yeast-bound form combined with vitamins A, C and E. After a few weeks his hip became much more mobile and both his day and night pain disappeared. The Arthritic Association decided to set up a trial, in 1982, and offered participation to 100 patients — the only proviso being that they were suffering seriously from arthritis. No attempts were made to diagnose differentially the exact type of arthritis. The results were a round endorsement of this selenium product with 70 per cent of the group reporting considerable improvement.

Another group of patients, this time rheumatoid arthritis patients who were shown to have low levels of selenium in their blood, were given selenium and vitamin E. The major result was pain reduction in a large number of the group. These trials were not of the 'double blind cross over' trial design favoured by doctors today, but such trials are in progress at the time of writing. Doctors understandably put much importance on these 'blind' trials (where neither doctor nor patient knows who is getting the test drug or an inert substance) because it is then possible to rule out the placebo response that so bedevils uncontrolled trials.

One way to eliminate the placebo response is to carry out animal trials, and this was done quite recently in the Animal Research Laboratory at the Boston City Hospital on a group of severely arthritic dogs and 70 per cent of these animals improved considerably on a regime of selenium and vitamin E.

Perhaps the largest trial to date has been, once again, an uncontrolled trial sponsored by *Here's Health* magazine. One thousand readers participated and a favourable response was noted in 90 per cent of the participants.

When one considers the very variable group of self-selected rheumatic sufferers that took part in these trials whose 'rheumatism' was a mixture of several rheumatic diseases, it is amazing that results of therapy were in any way favourable. After all, osteoarthritis ('wear and tear' rheumatism) is such a very different disease from rheumatoid arthritis with its auto-immune aetiology. But all rheumatisms involving joints do, when they reach the painful stage, involve the synovial membrane. This is exactly where masses of white cells gather and produce the joint damage that is characteristic of so much rheumatism. In all rheumatism at this painful stage the white cells are producing oxidants seemingly in an attempt to fight infection from germs (that do not exist). They do this by the production of superoxide radicals in excessive quantities.

It seems likely that selenium and other nutrients like vitamins A, E and C bring about their friendly effects by free radical 'scavenging'. And it is tempting to postulate that if these substances were present in the tissues in adequate quantities much rheumatism would be prevented. On-going research will doubtless eventually add further to our knowledge of how selenium helps with rheumatism. In the meantime there seems to be a wealth of evidence that selenium is Nature's own safe and gentle anti-inflammatory agent. Better rheumatism management without drugs and side-effects may well be just around the corner and based on selenium and other free radical scavengers.

One of the very latest developments in the management of rheumatoid arthritis was highlighted at the Third International Symposium on Selenium Biology and Medicine in Peking in 1984 and was a Japanese development pioneered by Dr Masaru of the Research Institute for Biological Ageing in Tokyo. It involved injecting rheumatoid arthritis victims with white blood cells donated by healthy young people, together with the administration of a selenium/yeast plus vitamin E preparation. Dr Masaru had previously found that remission of symptoms occurred in one patient in 30 who are given healthy white cells alone, but that if a selenium/yeast plus vitamin E product was given as well as the white cell injection a very high rate of remission, even in longstanding cases of rheumatoid arthritis, occurred.

CHAPTER 7
How selenium spares the heart

In Chapter 1 we met Dr Klaus Schwartz 'the man with a dream'. Dr Schwartz was, together with a handful of colleagues, the first to discover the essentiality in human nutrition of three trace elements chromium, fluorine and selenium. He told his wife Joyce Ann about his dream and it was an extremely worthy one. It was to eradicate at least one disease as a result of his scientific endeavours. Many doctors have had this Martin Luther King-type dream. Only a handful have seen it succeed, the Jenners and Salks of this world whose work eradicated smallpox and polio for instance. And of course there are others. But Dr Schwartz succeeded too — and in his own lifetime although few have read his story and know of his success.

Dr Schwartz's research on the essentiality of selenium was responsible for the elimination of a disease that you will not find very much about in medical books in the west. In fact it was a disease that has been endemic in China for many generations and is well documented in that country. It is called Keshan disease and it occurred widely in the area called the Mianning district of China where the disease was quite common prior to 1974. But by 1977 Keshan disease had been eradicated, thanks to the discovery of Klaus Schwartz.

Although young pregnant women were known to suffer from Keshan disease it was most prevalent in babies and small children where it presented as a very special form of heart failure. As it happens, it is not easy to diagnose heart failure in children, especially in country districts where diagnostic facilities are poor. Children with Keshan disease were mainly characterized by a failure to thrive. Mothers noticed that their babies gained weight very slowly, were often pale and would sweat a lot, and they lost weight easily too if they caught a chill or a cold. At feeding time such babies were irritable due to a frustrated desire to satisfy hunger quickly in the face of lack of energy and strength. A doctor examining such a child would note that his little heart was racing. He might be breathing over-fast too. Often, to start with, a simple feeding problem seemed the most likely diagnosis. But it would also be noted that such babies often looked pot-bellied and, on careful examination, the liver would be found to be enlarged — often considerably so.

Older children suffering from Keshan disease would tire easily. They would tend to get breathless on exertion. Often they would suffer a hacking cough and their neck veins would seem over-prominent. Their tummies would seem to bulge, and legs and feet would tend to swell at times. Such infants and children were often eventually diagnosed as suffering from heart failure only when they were near to death.

The commonest cause of heart failure in babies and small children throughout the whole world is congenital heart disease. But these Chinese children had none of the well-recognized signs of any of the several forms of congenital heart disease, and when children with Keshan disease died and their hearts were examined at autopsy there were no signs of any of the common anatomical defects seen in the hearts of congenital heart disease victims. Instead it was obvious that the cardiac muscle, that powers the heart, was abnormal. In fact it showed changes that resembled a disease that kills pigs. Widely spread in the myocardium (heart muscle) of children dying of Keshan disease were abnormal red patches which a fanciful veterinary surgeon, who first described the pig disease, thought resembled the fruits of the mulberry tree. Anyway he christened the condition Mulberry Disease. Significantly we now know that mulberry disease only afflicts pigs raised on selenium deficient diets.

———— Medical geography strikes again ————

When the medical geographers got to work in China they discovered a definite low-selenium-soil belt running from the north east to the south west of China. The Mianning country is set in the middle of this area. In 1974, when the facts about selenium began to be published, 4,510 children, selected randomly, were started on selenium supplements. Another random group of 3,985 children were selected as controls and were given a non-active placebo 'supplement'. In the following year as the scheme got going these groups were increased slightly to 6,709 and 5,445 children respectively. Two years later the results were so dramatically in favour of the selenium group that it was considered no longer ethical to carry on with the control group and all the children were given selenium.

In actual fact, during the first year of the trial 1.35 per cent of the control group developed Keshan disease as opposed to 0.22 per cent of the selenium supplement group. When the control group of the community was abolished and 12,579 children were all taking selenium supplementation the incidence of Keshan disease fell to 0.03 per cent. Selenium supplementation has now become mandatory in the area and during the last year that has been monitored no fresh cases of the disease have occurred. Dr Klaus Schwartz's dream had come true!

The fact that Keshan disease seems to be limited to China is, of course, very interesting and poses fascinating queries about the whole spectrum of trace element-deficiency disease that medical science has been slow to answer. Although soil, and therefore crop, selenium is very low in parts of China the same applies to elsewhere in the world where Keshan disease does not affect the children. It could be that children, and especially babies, live on a very restricted diet in this part of the world and therefore cannot gain even a trace of the essential selenium their hearts need. Or it could be that something that plays a large part of their normal diet interferes with their selenium absorption. This sort of phenomenon is common in trace element biology.

Keshan-type cardiomyopathy (heart-muscle disease) is common in intensively reared poultry, and it used to account for enormous losses of revenue to livestock rearers until selenium was added as a dietary supplement by poultry breeders in the USA.

At least one type of Keshan-type disease has occurred in the West and under very special circumstances. Two patients who were being fed parenterally (intravenously by drip feeding) with intravenous foodstuff suddenly and inexplicably developed heart failure. The accounts of the effects of selenium on Keshan disease had just been published in the *Lancet* and the doctors concerned added selenium to the parenteral feed. Incredibly quickly these patients' hearts recovered their normal action.

Not only a 'China syndrome'

In this country we do not see Keshan disease killing our children through severe lack of selenium. But there is an increasing weight of evidence becoming available that selenium can be, generally speaking, cardio-protective. But before we explore this in a little more detail it is necessary once again to try to get to grips with a problem that we all face. In other words why has heart disease and heart attack become so very much more prominent as a killer and spoiler of lives in the age in which we live?

How selenium spares the heart

The experts, the cardiologists, and our general practitioners all stress that heart disease is a very varied illness and is changing all the time. It can be caused by diseased valves in the heart. For example the valvular disease of the heart that was once so commonly caused by rheumatic fever is nowadays not the killer of young and middle-aged people that it was when I was a medical student. This is largely because penicillin prevents rheumatic fever complicating septic sore throats. Then there's heart failure that is secondary to other medical conditions, for example long and neglected chest disease or high blood pressure. But by far the most common heart disease today is due to diseases of the arteries, usually the arteries that actually feed and oxygenate the heart muscle itself, these are the coronary arteries that wind their way around the heart like a corona or crown. It is these vital arteries that the changes, known as atherosclerosis, occur that are capable of breeding blood clots or narrowing the arteries so much that the heart muscle cannot get enough oxygen. It is these diseased arteries that also cause the pain of angina and unpleasant illness of coronary thrombosis.

Not only do doctors quite rightly stress the various varieties of heart disease — they are also quite decided about some of the things that predispose us to heart disease. Some of these aetiological factors, to use the medical jargon, are very well established. Smoking has been proved so convincingly to be a prime example of an avoidable factor in heart and artery disease that nobody can argue against it.

Other common factors associated with the incidence of coronary artery disease are more complex and less easy to be dogmatic about. Medical geography has a strange story to tell in this instance, for it is possible to link the incidence of heart attack to selenium intake. But clearly other factors play a part as well. Two large population studies have linked fish-eating and the liability of developing heart attack. In two countries, Greenland and Japan, there is an enviably low rate of atheromatous disease evident and relatively few people die of coronary thrombosis. In both countries the population eat a lot of fish. Of course fish is relatively rich in selenium, although not in a particularly available form. In this country we do not eat much fish, in fact fish consumption has decreased by over 85 per cent in the last 100 years and it seems that this might be a factor worth considering when we consider why we are so coronary-prone in these islands.

The health in fish

Leaving aside fish as one of the world's great natural reservoirs of selenium, it seems likely that another factor in fish is also responsible for its protective action on the heart. This is the marine oil (or if you prefer it the fish fat) content of fish.

Recent reports have stressed the ways in which we must change our patterns of eating if we are to change from the top league members in the coronary death club to more enviable fourth division 'players' like the eskimos and the fish-eaters of Japan. One way is to radically change the *type* of fat we eat and to reduce the amount of hard fat (animal fat including milk products like butter and cheese) and to eat much more marine-based fat (like oily fish e.g. mackerel, salmon, sardines, pilchards and herrings) or to take oily fish dietary supplements.

You will notice that I have not mentioned polyunsaturates! Without going into masses of boring organic chemistry it is impossible to explain this controversy sensibly. In a nutshell, what is needed is less *animal* fat of all sorts in our diet and more *marine*-based fat which is rich in a fish-derived fatty acid called eicosapentaenoic acid or EPA for short. If we all designed our eating with this in mind we should all reduce our risk of coronary heart disease.

Selenium and the heart

Dr Raymond Shamberger of the Cleveland Clinic and Dr Johan Bjarksten of the Bjarksten Foundation were the first physicians to suggest that selenium might also have a profound effect on arteriosclerotic heart disease — the disease that is so closely implicated not only in coronary thrombosis but in stroke illness and high blood pressure. Now it would seem that selenium and EPA may well work together as cardioprotective substances in the following way.

A diet rich in EPA makes the blood clot much more slowly than it does if we eat masses of animal fat. (In fact dentists in Greenland loathe to extract the teeth of their Eskimo patients because so many of them bleed profusely after a dental extraction has been effected). Now, of course, blood that clots very slowly is clearly very useful when it comes to escaping a coronary thrombosis.

The selenium effect, however, would seem to be occurring actually in the artery wall rather than in the blood. It has been known for years that hard patches (doctors call them plaques) occurring on the inside surface of arteries are the starting points where the deadly clots form

1. NORMAL ARTERY

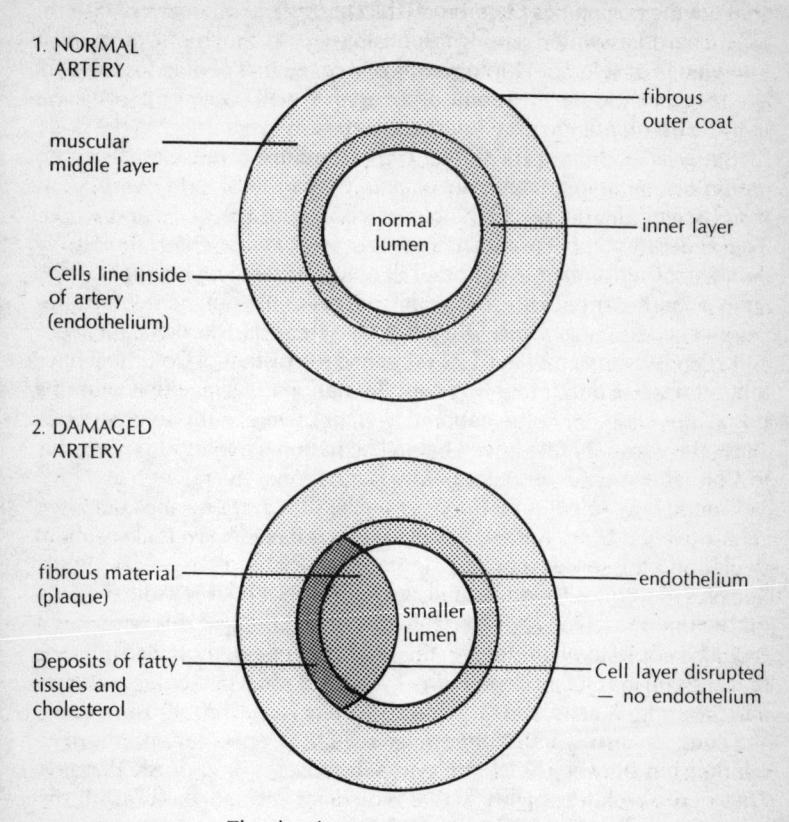

- fibrous outer coat
- muscular middle layer
- normal lumen
- inner layer
- Cells line inside of artery (endothelium)

2. DAMAGED ARTERY

- fibrous material (plaque)
- endothelium
- smaller lumen
- Deposits of fatty tissues and cholesterol
- Cell layer disrupted — no endothelium

The development of atheroslerosis

The first stage in atherosclerosis involves damage to the endothelial lining. The normal response to such damage — which occurs most readily at points of stress or turbulence — is for platelets to adhere to the area, covering and protecting it whilst it is repaired. In atherosclerosis this process fails to self-limit. If blood pressure is high both platelets and lipids infiltrate the inner layer, beneath the endothelium, and release chemicals which induce smooth muscle cells to migrate from the middle to the inner layer of the vessel. The narrowing of the arteries is irreversible and there is some loss of elasticity and the process continues and may be complicated by becoming the focus of a thrombosis, which further narrows the lumen.

that are the beginnings of coronary thrombosis and other artery disease. Dr Richard Passwater, who is responsible for so much of our modern knowledge of selenium biology, was one of the first people to point out the fact that the starting point of an arterial wall patch or plaque was in the muscular tissue that is part and parcel of every artery in the body. (If the arteries did not have their own little built-in muscles then they would not be able to 'open up' or 'shut down' the blood flow to allow for efficient circulation of the blood, cooling of the body and so on.) The Federation of American Societies for Experimental Biology in Anaheim, California, have probed deeply into medical geography and shown that Americans living in the selenium-deficient states of Connecticut, Illinois, Ohio, Oregon, Massachusetts, Rhode Island, New York, Pennsylvania, Indiana, Delaware and the district of Columbia have a heart disease death rate way over the national average (in Columbia it is 22 per cent above the national average), while in the selenium-rich states the coronary rate is well below the national average (for example in Colorado it is 67 per cent below the national average).

Exactly how selenium influences the health of arteries has not been exhaustively proved. But animal experiments have shown that selenium depletion causes vascular muscle damage. Richard Passwater clearly believes that this is fundamentally brought about by free radical attack on the tiny muscle in the arterial wall. Once damaged this becomes a focus for cholesterol infiltration, the beginning of a pathological process that ends up in calcium deposition — a state of affairs that makes arteries narrow and inelastic and which also fosters local thrombosis.

There is also some interesting scientific speculation about a relationship between selenium and substances called prostaglandins. These are the latest highly active biological substances to catch the attention of doctors and scientists. Originally discovered in extracts of the prostate gland, prostaglandins occur in many specific forms and are widely implicated in almost every type of biological tissue and pathological function. Essentially they seem to function as locally produced tissue hormones.

Generally speaking hormones are chemical messengers produced in specialized glands throughout the body that produce an effect *elsewhere* in the body. For instance, thyroid hormone produced in the thyroid gland in the neck controls the rate at which we burn up, or metabolize, food to produce energy. The pituitary gland, a tiny gland in the centre of our skull, produces all sorts of regulating hormones controlling things like growth rate and hormones that affect the sex glands, for instance the ovaries. These endocrine glands, as they are called, secrete their hormones *directly* into the bloodstream in which they are transported around the body. The hormone-like chemicals we call prostaglandins are made and act very locally in the body. A prostaglandin involved with digestion, for instance, is made and acts in the stomach. Another involved with the function of the womb originates in that organ.

Dr J. E. Vincent of the Department of Pharmacology at the Erasmus University believes that selenium deficiency is associated with a prostaglandin called E_2 which has an effect on blood clotting. He also feels that prostaglandin E_2-deficiency is incriminated in the whole process of atherosclerosis, and so a link is formed pretty directly between selenium deficiency, stroke illness and other cardiovascular problems of an arterial nature.

It cannot be claimed that this potential function of selenium has been extensively investigated in clinical trials. It did, however, form the subject of a medical thesis submitted to University of San Nicolas de Hidalgo in Morelia in Mexico a little over a decade ago in which a selenium/vitamin E combination product was used in a two-year trial with patients suffering from arteriosclerotic heart disease. It demonstrated improved cardiac function and a reduction in angina as well as a normalization of the ECG tracings in these patients.

And so we can say, without fear of contradiction, 'selenium spares the heart'. Exactly how beneficial it can be awaits the results of more trials and clinical research.

CHAPTER 8
Cancer prevention and selenium

There are all sorts of ways of preventing cancer. Nobody will argue about most of them. There is no doubt in any thinking person's mind that if you do not smoke cigarettes, for instance, you will be very unlikely to get cancer of the lungs. This is because you stop 'insulting' the cells that line the respiratory tract by coating them with tar every day of their lives. For years before we knew for certain how lung cancer originated scientists were aware that if you paint a rabbit's ear with tar every day it will eventually develop cancer of the ear due to chronic tar irritation.

Scientists in the 'tar ear-painting business' found out another fact about cancer while they were involved in these messy and unkind experiments. Some strains of rabbits got their cancer quite quickly; others took much more tar and time before the disease showed. In other words, there is a *genetic* factor at work that either predisposes us towards cancer or protects us against the dreaded disease.

Not all the cancer-causing factors that we know about are chemical ones, like tobacco. But we do know that there is an increasingly long list of chemical substances that produce cancers in folk who are exposed to them for any length of time, and public health measures are directed towards the protection of workers on this score wherever a sophisticated public health type of medical service is in operation.

Another type of preventable cancer is sunshine-induced skin cancer. President Reagan's experiences on this score are linked to his years in the saddle in California's semi-constant sunshine. In countries like Australia and other high ultra-violet light areas of the world sun worship has to be paid for in the penance that is skin cancer.

Another form of preventable cancer is cancer of the neck of the womb in women. This presents another interesting illustration of cancer prevention in action. Routine cervical screening in which a few cells are scraped from the neck of the womb, and examined under a microscope, sometimes demonstrates changes in the cells that cover the neck of the womb. These very early pre-cancerous changes in cells are harbingers of subsequent cervical cancer. When these are discovered as a *carcinoma in situ*, as it has been named, it is easy to 'peel' the neck of the womb surgically, just like you peel an apple, and remove these dangerous threatening cells and so obviate the cancer risk.

But now we know *why* these womb neck cells turn nasty in some women. It is due to an infection with a herpes-type virus. This virus is introduced into the woman's vagina by a man who himself has a herpes infection, or perhaps who carries that infection. It used to be unfairly said (mainly because cervical cancer never occurs in nuns) that female sexual activity and promiscuity were the basic cause of cervical cancer. Now we know that this is not so and, in fact, it is multiple sexual partner activity on the part of the male of the union that unhappily puts all his sexual partners at risk of developing cervical cancer.

But a huge range of cancers plague our world of which the basic cause is unknown or only partly known. For instance, we know that some cancers are influenced by dietary habits. Communities who traditionally exist on a very high-fibre diet rarely develop bowel cancer, for instance. In other cancers we have to rely on early diagnosis to give us the best choice of avoiding cancer and the breast self-examination schemes and mammography schemes are well-known examples of this very effective type of cancer avoidance and limitation.

Certain cancers show signs that we are winning the fight against malignant disease. For instance, 20 years ago cancer of the testes was almost certainly a sentence of early death for the victim. Today chemotherapy offers high cure rates. But in other cancers we have made only slight inroads into the cruel mass of disease that kills and maims thousands at all ages in all communities. Even if all the successes of cancer avoidance through not smoking or not coming into contact with any known cancer-producing agents are lumped together as success stories there still remains an awful lot of cancer that somehow flourishes and kills.

Selenium and cancer protection

The idea that selenium might act as a prophylactic against cancer sprang from relatively small beginnings. Dr Gerhard Schrauzer of the University of California in San Diego decided to see what effects selenium supplementation to the diet would have on a strain of mice that were known to be genetically liable to develop breast cancer quite frequently. About 83 per cent of such animals develop breast cancer during their natural lifespan. Selenium supplementation reduced this incidence to around 10 per cent! Subsequent work carried out at the Tumour Institute in Houston, Texas, also showed that selenium dietary supplementation reduced cancer incidence, a fact already known by sheep farmers in selenium-deficient New Zealand who found that by supplementing sheep fodder with selenium they could reduce the numbers of gastro-intestinal cancers in their sheep.

Medical geography produced the early indications that soil selenium, and its mirror image crop selenium, had a close relationship to breast cancer incidence too.

Drs Shamberger and Frost published a very interesting story on this score in the *Journal of the Canadian Medical Association* that showed that when crop selenium dipped below 0.05 parts per million, the breast cancer rate compared to average was raised by 9 per cent. But once the crop selenium rose to over 0.10 parts per million the breast cancer rate went down to only 20 per cent of the average. Further research along these lines investigated general cancer death rates among men, too, in areas of differing soil selenium levels.

Wherever the soil selenium was relatively high, that is over 0.26 parts per million in the soil, cancer rates were relatively low (392 per 100,000 death rate). In low soil selenium areas (between 0.01 and 0.05 parts per million) cancer rates were considerably increased (516 per 100,000 deaths).

Other studies in selenium medical geography confirm that the amount of selenium in the *blood* influences the chance we all have of suffering from cancer. In Rapid City in South Dakota, USA, they have the lowest recorded incidence of cancer in the United States — they also have the highest blood selenium levels. In Lima in Ohio where the cancer rates are twice those recorded in Rapid City, the blood selenium level sags at 60 per cent of the South Dakota level.

Of course, these two isolated instances are meaningless on their own. It could be that pollution levels, genetic factors or even different social habits between these two communities are responsible for these very interesting reports. Clearly Drs Shamberger and Willis of the Cleveland Clinic Foundation in the United States, who carried out this research, thought deeply on this possibility and went ahead and examined the cancer death rates in 19 cities scattered throughout the United States.

As a result they were able to produce a league table that directly related blood selenium measured in mcg per 100ml of blood to the cancer death rate that demonstrated an impressive relationship between blood levels of selenium and the cancer death rate per 100,000 of the population. Drs Schrouser, White and Schneider went even further in the exploration of the world of medical geography and produced a graph in a scientific journal (*Biorganic Chemistry*) that related annual selenium intake to age-corrected breast cancer death rates per 100,000 population in 29 countries throughout the world. It demonstrated an uncanny relationship between dietary selenium and the chance of dying of breast cancer. For example, in the UK and in Denmark the rate of death from breast cancer is about 24 per 100,000 of the population and in these countries the total amount of selenium intake is between 62 and 70mgs per person. In Taiwan and Japan where the death rate for breast cancer hovers around 3 and 4 per 100,000 women the annual selenium intake is around 85mgs per person per year.

Interest among doctors in Britain that selenium intake might well be related to your chance of dying of malignant disease (cancer) received a tremendous boost in 1983 when the prestigious medical journal *The Lancet* published a fascinating scientific report that hailed from the Harvard School of Public Health and the Johns Hopkins School of Hygiene and Public Health in conjunction with several other 'blue chip' medical centres in the US. This showed that the level of selenium circulating in the blood could be used as a sort of cancer diagnostic test. This study was conducted in such a way that it ruled out the possibility of factors other than selenium influencing results, and it involved a group of over ten thousand men and women who were being followed up on a large hypertension (high blood pressure) follow-up programme over several years. In a nutshell, it involved comparing the amount of selenium in the blood of 111 patients who developed cancer during a period of five years with the selenium level in the blood of 210 people in the survey who were cancer-free over the same period and who were matched for age, race, sex and even smoking history with the cancer victims. The mean blood selenium levels in the cancer group were significantly lower than in the cancer-free controls. The risk of cancer in the lowest quintile of blood selenium was twice that of the highest level. The association between low blood selenium and cancer was strongest for gastro-intestinal cancer and prostate gland cancer. Strangely, too, it was found that low levels of vitamins A and E compounded the effects of low blood selenium.

Groups of doctors and nutritional scientists of the calibre that took part in this impressive study are not prone to issue dramatic or overdrawn conclusions when their results are published, so they were at pains to point out that there was a possibility that their results were spurious. The risk of this being the case was minimal they felt, and went on to conclude that *low* selenium intake *increases* the risk of cancer and that additional selenium could benefit populations with low selenium intake. They also concluded that the mass of animal experiments in this field of study apply also to human beings.

——Where *The Lancet* leads others will follow——

If you, like me, are a 'chronic journal watcher' you will find that in almost any field of scientific research once one of the 'top flight' or 'blue chip' journals publishes a scientific or medical paper it somehow or other encourages others (with perhaps more nervous editors) to start publishing research projects that link into the general scheme of things, either positively or negatively. Quite soon after the previous 'cancer diagnosis' paper was published a group of workers from the Central Hospital in Kainuu, in Finland, published an account in the journal called *Carcinogenesis* that compared the blood selenium levels of 40 patients with cancer of the ovary (a particularly nasty form of cancer) with a series of age, weight and place-of-residence matched controls. The patients with cancer had a much lower blood selenium level (at a significant $p<0.001$ level) than controls.

This study also demonstrated that levels of blood selenium followed the outcome of the disease. In other words blood selenium increased as patients got better or decreased as they deteriorated. The authors of this fascinating study emphasized that Finland increased the amount of imported (higher selenium content) cereals during 1980 and 1982, and in that period the dietary intake of selenium approximately doubled. During this period the remission rate from this unpleasant disease increased significantly too.

Quite soon after this article was published in *Carcinogenesis* another significant report appeared — this time from one of the most prestigious cancer research centres in the USA, the Sloan-Kettering Center in New York. This was an animal study that demonstrated that selenium decreased the incidence of artificially induced cancer of the large bowel of rats. A mixture of well-known carcinogens (cancer inducers) was given to groups of rats some of which were given selenium-fortified drinking water at the same time. This selenium 'drink' delayed the subsequent development of cancer of the colon and more so in the 'proximal' parts of the colon than in 'distal' parts.

——More interest in colon cancer and selenium——

Cancer of the large bowel is one of the commonest forms of cancer in humans and 4 per cent of us have a lifetime risk of developing this disease. Shortly after the previous Sloan-Kettering 'rat' paper was published, a journal called *Disease of the Colon and Rectum* published a paper from the Department of Surgery, Illinois Hospital in Chicago. This put forward the hypothesis that the increasing incidence of this type of cancer was owing to deficiency of selenium in the blood through decreased consumption of selenium in the diet. It also suggested that selenium absorption was adversely affected by an increased zinc fluoride content in the diet. Dr Richard L. Nelson, who wrote this article, suggested that a high zinc dietary intake was related to the increased meat consumption in the USA which has risen by 50 per cent in the last 30 years (and incidentally by 100 per cent in the UK).

Zinc from meat sources is known to prevent the absorption of selenium, and has been demonstrated to be capable of abolishing selenium's protective effects in experimental animal studies.

——Womb cancer and selenium protection——

As mentioned previously, at least one form of womb cancer (cervical cancer) is virus-induced and largely preventable through the procedure known as cervical screening (PAP testing) and by the modification of sexual behaviour. Cancer of the main body of the womb (endometrial cancer) is not either virus-induced or related to sexual behaviour. A research study has been carried out at Oula University in Finland and reported in the *International Journal of Gynaecology and Obstetrics*. It involved over 100 mixed womb cancer patients aged between 37 and 83 years and showed that they had a singificantly ($P<0.001$) lower blood selenium level than a control group that were age, weight and location matched.

Once again the research staff, after drawing attention to evidence that patients with a wide variety of cancers (including gastro-intestinal cancer, Hodgkin's disease, chronic lymphatic leukaemia, and breast cancer) have lower blood selenium than do control patients. It was also pointed out, sagely, that low blood selenium might be a *contributing factor* in the *development* of the cancer rather than being the *result of the illness*.

Later in the year (1984) the *American Journal of Epidemiology* addressed itself to the question of levels of selenium in the blood, and the development of cancer generally, in a study carried out at the University of Kuopio, again in Finland, where a population of over 8,000 men and women, aged from 31 to 59 were monitored over a six-year period. All the study group were initially free of cancer. Controls were carefully matched according to age, sex, daily tobacco consumption and their serum cholesterol level. The results of this exhaustive study showed a strong association between low serum selenium and cancer risk. The intake of selenium of those in this study was low (about 20 micrograms per day).

The *BMJ* stands up to be counted

The *British Medical Journal* is the mouthpiece and reflection of informed medical comment in Britain and speaks with a degree of informed comment that is unique in the world of medical science. Each week the *BMJ* receives an enormous postbag of scientific and medical papers 'for favour of publication'. The majority of these are rejected by the editor and his staff. A small proportion are provisionally accepted by the editor and promptly sent off to medical 'referees' — all eminent medical people who are often specialists in their field. Once again they reject a fair proportion of the papers sent to them or suggest they are returned to the authors for amendment or clarification. Eventually the favoured few of the mass of articles go for 'hanging'. This means that once a week a further group of 'Friends of the journal' peruse this *crême de la crême* and once again accept or reject them. As a result the *British Medical Journal* only contains a very well selected series of articles that have passed perhaps the most strenuous medical scrutiny that it is possible to arrange.

One such article published in 1985 came once again from Finland, a country that as well as labouring under low soil-selenium is also, for various social reasons, peculiarly well suited to carrying out large population studies on its people. The particular study that won the *BMJ*'s seal of clinical approval studied 51 case control patients, that is 51 patients and 51 others paired with a control-matched person (for age, sex and smoking) which came from a random sample of some 12,000 people aged 30-64 years.

Cancer prevention and selenium

When the study was complete, it was demonstrated that patients who died of cancer during the follow-up period had a 12 per cent lower blood selenium level than did their matched controls. In this study, blood concentrations of vitamins A and E were also examined. The data collected after analysis showed that those subjects in the lowest tertile of blood selenium concentration had a 5.8 times greater risk of developing cancer than did controls. If their vitamin E blood level was also low this risk grew to 11.4 times. In smokers with cancer, the vitamin A level in the blood was 26 per cent lower than in smoker controls, so clearly decreased vitamin A increases the risk of lung cancer in men with a low selenium intake.

Once again the eminent medical men or women who carried out this important study at the University of Kuopio in Finland draw very circumspect conclusions. As the *BMJ* reports:

> Owing to the design of our study we cannot rule out the possibility that serum concentrations of the substances measured were not the truly protective factors but merely indicators of other compounds or nutrients that were the real causal factors. Nevertheless, other studies and our findings indicate that dietary selenium deficiency increases the risk of cancer, possibly irrespective of site, and that this effect is enhanced by a low vitamin E intake. Furthermore, a decreased intake of β carotene or retinol (vitamin A) or both seems to contribute to the risk of lung cancer among smoking men with a low intake of selenium.

As might be expected the research team advise more research on this particularly important subject. For my money, and I suspect most doctors would agree with me, from the practical point of view the whole matter is proved beyond reasonable doubt and the main problem to be solved is exactly what must we do about it.

—Looking at the whole problem in perspective—

It must by now be glaringly obvious that medical science has, in the matter of selenium, to make enormously important decisions as far as the avoiding of cancer is concerned. Are we to make a conscious effort to increase our daily intake of selenium in the way of including more selenium-rich food in our regular eating habits? Or should we perhaps cut down on foodstuffs that tend to prevent selenium absorption, like meat? Should we take a daily selenium supplement, or should we sweep all the available scientific evidence we have been looking at under the carpet and pretend it does not exist? Strangely, perhaps, the medical establishment, together with most of the media, tends to incline to supporting the latter view at the moment.

It is interesting perhaps that when non-clinical research workers approach this problem they often seem to come up with a more positive view on the subject. A preview of the part that nutrients can play in cancer protection was recently reported in *Perspectives in Practice* (1986) by the Department of Family and Community Medicine in the Arizona Health Sciences Center in Tucson, USA. It was supported by a National Cancer Institute grant. It concluded that:

> It has been estimated that 35 per cent of all cancer incidence is related to diet. The potential appears great that high intakes of various nutrients can reduce the incidence of some types of cancer. Selenium and vitamins A, C and E, discussed in this article, have many actions and interactions that are important in relationship to the study of nutrition and cancer. Even though only a few of the necessary human trials of efficacy have been conducted, epidemiological and animal data suggest that vitamins and/or minerals act as anti-carcinogens, altering cancer incidence, differentiation, and growth. Thus, they may prove useful adjuncts to conventional therapies or in cancer prevention. However, the nutrients should not be viewed as cure-alls that work alone. Adequate intake ideally should be the result of increased dietary consumption rather than supplements because as yet unidentified components found in food may prove beneficial and protective. More research is needed prior to encouraging members of the general population to increase their intakes of various nutrients, even though there is now some evidence that those nutrients may help some cancers.

There is undoubtedly a deal of sense in what these workers in Arizona have to say about the importance of making changes in eating practices rather than turning to the simpler solution of taking a dietary supplement as a selenium insurance policy with cancer protection in mind; provided, that is, that first of all domestic or commercial food processing of our selenium-rich food does not deplete it of the vital trace element it contains. From the practical point of view this can be very difficult, however, and daily selenium supplementation by those who fear death from cancer now seems a sensible precaution.

The final solution — Finnish style

Finland, as we have said, has like most of Scandinavia a very low concentration of selenium in her soil. The same applies to Great Britain, apart from East Anglia. Professor Pekka Koivistoinen of Helsinki University has recently reviewed the whole situation in Finland and outlined a novel way of solving the various health problems that accrue from this unfortunate state of affairs. The low soil selenium in Finland comes about because geochemically 60 per cent of the rock foundation upon which Finland lies is igneous in origin and contains little selenium. Much of the natural selenium health heritage was 'leached out' during the Ice Age. The Finnish climate with its low temperatures and relatively high humidity reduces soil selenium further and alters the composition of such selenium as does remain into a form that is poorly available to plants.

The Finns were one of the first nations in the world to relate their poor natural sources of selenium to a variety of ills and diseases in their farm animals and have been supplementing animal feeds with selenium since 1969.

During the 1970s the Finns were at pains to define the paucity of selenium in their food. They found that their drinking water contained virtually no selenium at all. The average intake in Finnish diet was about 25 micrograms per day. Finnish breast-fed babies did extremely badly as far as selenium was concerned, as their mothers' milk contained such low amounts that they obtained only 4.7 micrograms per day by the time they were 3 months old.

To start with, the Finns attempted to tackle their selenium deficiency by importing high selenium wheat and, indeed, by 1981 this had raised the average dietary intake to about 50 micrograms. They also observed the effect of selenium supplementation on a group of 'healthy' men who were known to have a low blood selenium to see whether selenium-rich wheat or a selenium supplement worked better. Both doubled the platelet glutathione activity — a reliable index of selenium absorption.

The Finnish agricultural and public health authorities were sufficiently worried about the long-term effects of their country's low soil-selenium and its effect on health that they drew up what might be thought of as a final solution to the problem. They decided to embark on a massive policy to 'put back' the selenium into the soil by adding selenium to fertilizers.

As from July 1984 all the NPK fertilizers used in Finland were 'fortified' with selenium at a concentration of either 6 or 16 mgs per kg. It is estimated that between 5 per cent and 30 per cent of the selenium applied to the soil finds its way into harvested crops, and it is aimed to elevate food crop selenium to more acceptable levels. The Finnish agriculturists realize fully that this is something in the nature of a 'last ditch' salvage operation. The accumulation of selenium in the soil will be very slow, and a doubling of soil selenium by this method would probably take 100 years. Nevertheless, this bold Finnish experiment is entirely laudable as the reaction of a relatively small country to the high heart disease and cancer rates that are inherent in having to live on a soil low in selenium.

To date there is no evidence of similar schemes being put into operation in selenium-deficient Britain or the USA.

CHAPTER 9
Escaping micronutrient failure

It would be marvellous if we knew *exactly* how micronutrients like selenium seem to help us escape getting crotchety with rheumatism or prevent us from developing heart disease. It would be doubly marvellous, if we knew, to some extent at least, how they can also seemingly instruct our biological ageing clocks to 'go easy'. To understand exactly how they seem to be protective against cancer would of course be quite fantastic.

It certainly seems likely that the 60 trillion or so cells that make up our bodies are constantly under attack from the free radicals that were mentioned in Chapter 5 but our bodies use some of these free radicals for quite proper and useful purposes. Somehow or other, though, free radicals may 'escape' and cause the damage we have been considering.

In the case of rheumatism it seems likely that these free radicals find themselves able to attack the joint cartilages and synovial membranes. Another way they attack us is via the cells that line the inner surfaces of our arteries and their muscular walls providing a little nest or *nidus* for arteriosclerosis to lodge in. It is also quite feasible that free radicals can 'home in' on the basic mechanisms of cell reduplication — the 'triple helix' of our hereditary birthright — and so disturb it that subtly abnormal cells are produced. Although 'foreign' in one way to our system these altered cells are not recognized as such by the body's normal defence mechanisms, and so escape to cause cancer.

There is a strong mass of evidence that the body uses certain nutritional substances, particularly vitamins A, C and E, often referred to as *antioxidants*, to mop up and redirect these free radicals, and selenium seems to work in precisely the same fashion. Several research workers, one of whom is Dr Douglas Frost of the Trace Mineral Laboratory in New York, have gone on record as saying that selenium and vitamin E work synergically, each helping the other to carry out this vital anti-oxidant free radical scavenging function.

Although there seems little chance of our proving it, there is considerable circumstantial evidence that free radical attack on all the cells of our body is very much involved in the ageing process, particularly causing the phenomenon of cross-linking, and there is a lot of sound biological evidence that certain nutrients are also effective, to some extent at least, in slowing down this cross-linking — particularly vitamins A, B_1, B_5, B_6, C, E and notably the mineral selenium.

When it comes down to asking 'why?' questions, relative to possible nutritional influences on various disease states, the victim of the illness under consideration often, and quite justifiably, asks: 'Why me? Why is it that, although I eat the same sort of food, have the same sort of lifestyle, take the same amount of exercise, enjoy the same amount of sleep, play as hard, relax as assiduously as you do — I get ill and you don't?' An easy and rather glib answer to this difficult question has been to point to genetic differences. But, other than in a handful or so of diseases, it is difficult to mount any serious defence of genetic differences having very much to do with why I get ill and you don't. And vice versa! In most cases it appears that an 'x' factor is operating that either gives or denies us protection. There is some evidence that the mystery 'x' factor may well lurk in the first few loops of our small intestine — a part of our inside that I like to call our *absorption organ*. It could be that what happens there has a greater effect on whether you or I get sick or stay well — especially as far as diseases related to nutritional trace elements are concerned — than anyone realizes.

The forgotten organ

The modern concept of the absorption organ has come about mainly as a result of intensive research carried out by a body of specialist doctors who call themselves gastroenterologists. For years they have been puzzling over the problem of why some people get nutritionally ill while eating a particular sort of diet when others don't. This problem is hardly new. In fact, medical history gives us examples going back to the beginning of the century if we look for them.

Way back in 1905 a physician working in villages in the foothills of the Himalayas noted that a certain proportion of the population developed neck tumours called goitres; and that cretinism, idiocy and deaf mutism were common there too. Another village nearby, that obtained water from a different source, did not suffer in this way. In the 1920s a doctor working in Akron, Ohio, USA, demonstrated that giving schoolgirls a small dose of iodine every day had a most beneficial result. This area, too, was notorious for a high incidence of goitre. As a result of a four-year experiment which involved 5,000 girls he proved that:

Of those taking iodine — if the girls were normal at the beginning of the experiment no goitres developed at the end of the experiment. If, however, they were goitrous at the beginning, two-thirds became normal.

Of the controls (not taking iodine) — if normal at the beginning of the four-year experiment 50 per cent became goitrous within four years. If any were goitrous at the beginning of the experiment none became normal in four years.

This type of nutritional goitre occurs everywhere in the world where water is deficient in the micronutrient iodine. It used to be very prevalent in the Pennines in this country where it gained the nickname of Derbyshire Neck. Today is it a rarity because the Ministry of Health several decades ago introduced the use of iodized table salt in the UK.

But the significance of these little bits and pieces of medical history and their relevance to the absorption organ has been slow to sink in, particularly to medical personnel. Not *all* the Indian villagers in the goitre area developed goitre. Not *all* the schoolgirls in Ohio had swollen necks. Although they *all* were taking in the same very small quantities of iodine, some had very efficient absorption organs that somehow managed to extract enough iodine to prevent a goitre even *from very low iodine water.*

Modern gastroenterologic research has busied itself of recent years in trying to solve many outstanding problems of food absorption. For instance there is a pretty rare but well-defined illness called Whipple's Disease (named after Dr Whipple, a distinguished American doctor from the Johns Hopkins Hospital in Baltimore) in which victims start to waste away, get diarrhoea, and suffer from glandular enlargement, that is caused by a disease process in parts of their absorption organ. There's another disease called Hartnup Disease in which a defect in the absorption organ prevents the efficient absorption of just one particular protein. It seems highly likely that inefficient absorption organs are the basic cause for many diseases related to selenium depletion.

—What's so special about the absorption organ?—
Well, to start with it's about the largest internal organ of the body (it is nine metres long). If we look inside it with a microscope, it looks like

a coral reef covered by a mass of sea anemones — each hungry for sustenance. In fact, the analogy has been drawn that developmentally its structure is a reminder that we once evolved from aquatic creatures getting our nutrients from whatever wafted past us on the waves!

If we look at these 'anemones' in more detail (they are called villi), by the side of each of these structures, that waves finger-like to its millions of fellows, there is a dent (or crypt). This little device increases the surface area of the organ. If we look at the villi through a high-powered microscope it will be noticed that inside each 'finger' there is a fine leash of blood vessels enmeshed in jelly-like substance. Nature has designed this structure so delicately that the nutrients in our absorption organ (the semi-digested food) are separated from our blood stream by the width of one single cell. And this is the precise point where you and I come into contact with things outside us (and in this case the food that we eat) most intimately. So intimately, indeed, that we can absorb it into our substance.

Some people have difficulty in taking this concept in. When we swallow food and it enters our digestive tract it really remains 'outside us'. It merely changes from being on your plate to being in a tube that is running through you enclosing a bit of the 'outside' as it were. It is only when, after digestion has converted food into a sort of nutritious soup, that the absorption organ 'sucks it in' as it were, into the tissues of you and me. (This is exactly the point, in fact, where, as the poet said, 'everything Miss T eats turns into Miss T.')

The 'second brain' concept

There is another fascinating side to the absorption organ that has been kept very quiet by doctors and scientists generally. But an eminent gastroenterologist writing in *The Journal of the Royal Society of Medicine* recently drew his fellow members' attention to the fact that in the absorption organ, and especially in its first part, within the glove-finger-like crypts there are masses of cells that take up a special stain for nervous tissue. Of course the whole of the gastro-intestinal tract needs nerves to provide the circuitry to make its muscles work and 'power along' the bowel contents. But the elaborate nerve complexity of the first few metres of the absorption organ is so very impressive and substantial that the term 'second brain' does not seem inappropriate.

It has been known for years now that certain psychological and even psychiatric problems are often associated with bowel symptoms. For instance, in anxious or nervous folk discomfort after eating is quite common, and such people will often complain of excessive bowel rumblings and 'wind'. In some cases this extends to a state of affairs in which there is a period of bloatedness and 'heaviness' of the bowel shortly after eating. Sometimes, too, there is a period several hours after eating during which there is a tendency towards over-action of the bowel. 'My inside works overtime', as one patient put it. This simple derangement of the absorption organ is so common these days that cases seem to be the major problem that gastro-intestinal clinics have to deal with in our hospitals. Recently this nervous complex of bowel dysfunction has been given a brand new name — the irritable bowel syndrome (IBS for short).

Doctors and specialists of every persuasion, general practitioners, physicians, surgeons, psychiatrists, alternative medicine practitioners and nutritionists have all puzzled over just why this new disease is with us, and all sorts of theories that range from allergy to food additives and stress have been put forward to try to explain the cause of the problem. From the point of view of our interest — the influence that trace elements generally, and selenium in particular, have in the prevention of a wide range of nasty diseases — the presence of the irritable bowel syndrome in all probability aggravates poor selenium absorption and explains to some extent why some folk can 'get away' with a low selenium diet while others get ill as a result.

A sluggish absorption organ

As you might expect there is every possible example of variations in absorption organ function, and it seems likely that these variations effect particularly the absorption of trace elements, which are by definition present in only minute quantities in the semi-digested 'soup' that passes through the bowel. We know that two mechanisms are involved in all absorption. Some substances simply flow into the villi and so on into the bloodstream in what is called a *concentration gradient system*. This works poorly for trace elements. Other substances seem to be actively sought out by the villi which need to expend vital bio-energy to 'pump' them into our system. We see this happening for instance in the great variation that occurs from person to person in the absorption of certain vitamins, like vitamin C. Really, medical history tells us this is so. In the old sailing ships, that were so long out at sea that they ran out of all fresh vegetables, not all the sailors developed scurvy although they all experienced the same lack of vitamin C in their diet. This was because some had absorption organs that were very efficient and really 'sucked up' every little bit of vitamin C available even in long-stored food. Others had organs that were less efficient.

Another way of proving this vast biological variation in the activity of the absorption organ has been mentioned earlier and is quoted by the world-famous nutritionalist Dr Jeffrey Bland in his book *Medical Applications of Clinical Nutrition* (Keats). Dr Bland points out that a very good way to decide when somebody is fully 'topped-up' with vitamin C is to measure the amount of vitamin C they have to swallow so that 50 per cent of this amount is excreted in the urine. In one test involving a group of nine normal adult women a variation of dosage of 0.6 to 2.2mg of vitamin C per kilogram of their body weight was necessary to reach this top-up level denoting a very considerable variation of their absorption organs' efficiency.

When we look at many of the diseases that we have been examining in this book — heart disease, rheumatism, cancer and so on — it is surprising how often doctors will state that a contributory factor, that seems to dictate to some extent whether or not patients develop disease, seems to be stress. Doctors and nutritionists who have spent years of their lives working on vitamins and nutrients to try to decide approximately what the recommended daily allowances of various nutritional substances are to keep us from developing deficiency symptoms have repeatedly drawn attention to the fact that stress alters RDAs. This stress may stem from an operation, an accident, or other sort of trauma, and it always means that the RDA must be increased if disease due to absorption efficiency is to be avoided. Drugs, including nicotine, alcohol and the Pill, as well as the vast array of medicines that some folk have to take, alter the absorption organ's function, too. It seems that all these factors operate by depressing the bio-energy of the cells of our absorption organ, which subsequently is depressed in its vital functioning. Selenium as a substance in low concentrations in our food is terribly vulnerable in this way.

Will dietary improvement help us to better absorption organ function?

To a certain extent dietary improvements will allow the absorption organ to function optimally *if* the diet contains a wide range of naturally-grown food (not commercially-grown crops on soils in which extensive artificial fertilizer boosting has allowed plants to 'leach out' vast quantities of micronutrients that Nature can never replace). A large proportion of any ideal diet should be eaten raw to obviate cooking degradation and vaporization of nutrients — especially selenium. When this diet is designed, purified sugars, milled grains, alcohol and saturated fat should be minimal in content unless three to four times standard RDA of most minerals and vitamins are added as diet supplements — including selenium.

—Boosting dietary selenium to improve health—

At the end of Chapter 3 there is a fairly exhaustive breakdown of the selenium content of most basic foods, and intelligent selection from this list can helpfully boost selenium intake. But always it is important to be aware of the fact that the real selenium content of foods is to some extent a matter of hopeful guesswork rather than precise fact. We all get the majority of our selenium from grain and grain products. But, of course, the *source* of the grain dictates the amount of selenium it contains. Grain from Finland, most of Scandinavia and Britain is poor as far as selenium content is concerned, and whenever grains are subjected to high temperatures the selenium content tends to be reduced as well.

This whole problem of bio-availability has to be taken into earnest consideration when we are contemplating the trace element content of food. Bio-availability really defines 'usability' of the substance under consideration, and so is involved in its *absorption* (how efficient is the absorption organ?), and its *transport* around the body (some sorts of selenium are more mobile in the body than others). It also directs itself to the question of the excretion of the substance in question (certain drugs stimulate mineral excretion, for instance diuretic pills). All these considerations are important.

For instance, Japan seems to do very well theoretically with a per capita selenium intake of 200 micrograms per day, that is until it is pointed out that the selenium in fish (Japan's main source of selenium) has a low bio-availability. It would appear that only a fraction of the total selenium in most fish, including tuna, herring and mackerel, is really available for biological purposes.

Another 'popular' source of dietary selenium is mushrooms, but only certain species contain a high content of selenium, and there is a species variation of between 0.01 and 37mg of selenium per kilo of various mushrooms! Unfortunately, most of the mushrooms in our shops and supermarkets are *Agaricus bisporus* and this has a poor selenium content. To some extent the content depends on the selenium content of the irrigation water used (like most plant sources of selenium) and it has been demonstrated that the selenium content of mushrooms of the *Agaricus bisporus* species can be increased up to eight times by suitable sodium selenite supplements.

The selenium content of certain meats is also substantial (on paper) but once again this depends on exactly *how* the animal is fed on the hoof, and is also depressed by general low bio-availability factors. In view of all these possible biological question marks many responsible nutritionists and physicians believe that the safest way to be sure that you are getting enough selenium is to take a selenium supplement.

CHAPTER 10

Feeling one degree under-and selenium

It is very difficult to get a heterogeneous group of people to agree about anything, and you cannot really get more heterogeneous than the medical profession. If ever you have been the centre of a medical debate about your own health you will know what I mean. Say, for instance, your general practitioner sends you to hospital because you develop something quite straightforward, like a hernia. The surgical specialist says: 'Fine, come to hospital and I will stitch it up for you!' But if as well as a hernia you also suffer another of the ills that flesh is heir to the problem can get complicated. Perhaps you have a diabetic condition, or bronchitis, in which case the physician responsible for your general medical condition may say: 'Hold on. I'm not sure it is a good idea for you to have an operation! Why not try a truss?' And so you tend to be tossed about a bit on the horns of a therapeutic dilemma and medical debate.

Now, the solution of this sort of problem really should be quite simple. After all, it deals with medical principles that are pretty stereotyped. But, when we get into areas of possible therapeutic controversy the great divide in medical thinking becomes much wider. We saw this in action recently in the UK with reference to the Alternative Medicine debate. Alternative Medicine has a straightforward following in Britain that is headed up by the very elite of our land. (The Royal Family are dedicated to homoeopathy, and Prince Charles quite clearly champions those who feel that an open mind on the claims of Alternative Medicine should be mandatory.) Strangely, perhaps, the British Medical Association was entrusted with an enquiry into Alternative Medicine. I say 'strangely' because the BMA represents the most conservative fraction of a very conservative profession in this matter, and their findings were naturally predictable.

One very common matter that doctors and patients tend to disagree about was, however, nothing to do with Alternative Medicine or the pros and cons of 'medical' versus 'surgical' treatment of hernias or anything else. It involves the curious state of ill-health that we all know exists but is so very difficult to define that we tend to describe it as being 'run-down'.

When this happens, all of a sudden everything seems an effort. A job that we usually can polish off in ten minutes takes half an hour. It is difficult to get up in the mornings and we tend to fall asleep in the evenings in front of the TV and miss our favourite programme! When this 'run-down' syndrome strikes it is tempting to postpone anything that we possibly can.

Sometimes doctors incline to the view that this 'run-down' problem is largely psychological, and there is indeed a form of depression that does present in this way. There is, however, a movement in the medical profession to reappraise this whole condition especially when, as well as the run-down symptomology, patients suffer the 'cold after cold' syndrome.

Now, we all get three to four colds a year, the symptoms of which last about a week, and the old adage that with medical treatment you can clear a cold in seven days, whereas if you leave it to Nature it can go on for a full week is undoubtedly true! But there's very definitely a minority of folk who really suffer the 'cold after cold' syndrome. No sooner does one cold clear than another one seems to set in. In a small minority of such cases it is possible to find a medically obvious reason for this state of affairs — a chronic sinus infection perhaps. But in the majority of cases nothing apart from the 'cold after cold' syndrome seems to be present.

It has been known both to mothers and all who care for small children that they, too, suffer from this 'cold after cold' problem, in which case the hallmark of the syndrome is chronic catarrh and poor appetite. For many years it was left to mothers to manage this problem as best they could, and indeed they often went to the chemist and bought a tonic for their children in the face of little help from their medical advisers. To everyone's delight, quite often this tonic worked dramatically. Doctors generally would mumble something about a 'placebo effect' or 'Nature at work' when this happened, that is until one doctor did a series of simple investigations on these catarrhal and sickly children and found, in fact, they were suffering from a nutritional deficiency — a deficiency of an oft-forgotten trace element, iron. What had happened in the case of the surprising response to the medicine from the chemist was that the tonic recommended was usually Minadex or a similar mixture — a well-known vitamin and iron supplement. Quite rapidly the children rebuilt their low stores of iron and their immune system got a boost allowing them to shrug off the infections that were laying them low.

A licence to survive

Although in adults iron deficiency is not an enormously important factor in producing the strange general debility that sends us off in search of a tonic or something to 'give us a boost' it does happen, particularly in women or girls who are cursed by over-heavy, over-long or over-frequent periods, and by those who because of religious or personal reasons are strict vegetarians.

A more likely reason for feeling 'one degree under', 'off colour' or 'permanently bushed' in the general run of people is some temporary malfunction of the immune system. The immune system was very effectively described by Dr Robert Good of the Sloan-Kettering Center for Cancer Research in the following phrase: 'Man lives in a sea of micro-organisms, the immune system is his license to survive.' The immune system is, like the 'second brain' we were involved with in the previous chapter, hidden away in our body. Sometimes you can 'feel it' struggling into activity when you get a short sharp attack of 'flu and your very bones ache as the white cells from your bone marrow are suddenly called for in large numbers.

Evidence that the immune system is there as your survival licence also shows when the glands in your throat and neck suddenly enlarge if tonsillitis strikes or you go down with an attack of glandular fever. All these things are encouraging signs that you are fighting for survival against bacterial or viral attack. But by far the main reaction is quite hidden unless somebody examines your blood biochemistry, in which case your lymphocytes, which are white cells derived from the lymph tissue (those enlarged glands), your macrophages, the large scavenger cells, and antibodies (largely chemical defences) can be demonstrated reacting to your plight.

There are several different types of lymphocytes. The so-called T cells seem to be the first wave of general assault troops against an invasion of the body. Sometimes they misfire, as we have seen in Chapter 6, and get involved in the production of the auto-immune diseases, almost by accident you might say. The B lymphocyte cells seem to be more involved in specific antibody formation. There are other cells which are concerned in this whole process, too. It seems that all these defence cells spring from a basic *stem cell* found in our bone marrow; they are the shock troops of your immune system — your passport to survival.

Selenium boosts the system

All sorts of things can depress the efficiency of the immune system. Radiation, toxic chemicals, certain viruses, like AIDS, and bacteria, stress and poor nutrition are a few common examples. A suggestion that micronutrient and vitamin deficiency could have a profound effect on the ability of the body to keep its defences well primed hailed from Soviet research way back in 1972. When immunologists are evaluating the efficiency of a vaccine they do so by measuring the level of antibody produced, either in the human or in a suitable laboratory animal, after an injected dose of antigen (the biological 'tag' by which the body recognizes the presence of a foreign invader). The Soviet scientist involved was working with a typhoid vaccine and found that he could get a much better 'antibody response' if, as well as the vaccine under test, he also gave selenium and vitamin E to his research animals.

In the following year scientists at Colorado State University duplicated this work and also showed that both antibody level and the number of antibody-producing cells could be enhanced in similar circumstances by supplements of selenium alone. What was more interesting still was that the immune response seemed to be dose-related. In this case they began by enriching sheep's diets by 0.7 parts of selenium per million. This produced a seven-times increase in antibody production after the antigen stimulus. If the dose of selenium was increased so that the diet contained 2.8 parts per million the antibody response was raised 30-fold, a reaction surely too specific to be some sort of biological accident.

Further animal research has confirmed this boosting facility of the immune response in a variety of animals including mice, guinea pigs and in experiments involving canine distemper vaccine in dogs. The most impressive real evidence that low blood selenium could bring about a poor biological (antigenic) response to the general run of invading organisms in humans had to wait until doctors started to investigate a very strange illness that struck down a whole host of people in the US at a Philadelphia convention in 1976.

The American Legion is a group of senior citizens, very much like our British Legion, with whom it shares similar aims. They hold group meetings and are involved in a variety of charitable works. At the particular meeting referred to, delegates fell ill in large numbers with a disease now called Legionnaire's Disease. It is characterized by abdominal pain, fever and a bad headache. Later pneumonia developed in many victims. Untreated, the illness was serious and had a mortality of 20 per cent.

Since this epidemic more than 20 outbreaks of Legionnaire's Disease have occurred all over the world, and the disease has strangely been 'pinned down', not to a droplet person-to-person infection like 'flu or colds, but to the inhalation of water vapour from showers and air-conditioning plants containing a bacterium that has been named *legionella pneumophilia* after the unfortunate first victims. One of the interesting findings in Legionnaire's Disease is that not everyone exposed to the infection develops the disease, and that in one group of 17 victims one abnormal finding in their blood was a low selenium content.

Clearly, we are here very much in the realm of supposition and *post hoc propter hoc* reasoning. Further research is needed to investigate the blood selenium status of those who feel themselves so 'run down' or 'off colour' that they take themselves off on a recuperative holiday, go to an expensive health farm or to a hydro where they part with large sums of money to eat masses of (selenium-rich) raw vegetables while eschewing such things as meat and saturated fat that are known to reduce the amount of selenium absorbed into the body. But some such folk will often go to the pharmacy in search of a tonic. If it is going to have a chance of really stimulating a flagging immune response it had better contain selenium and preferably vitamin A, E and C as well.

CHAPTER 11
Not only but also

Most interest in selenium's value as a micronutrient has been generated via the Health Food Industry both in Britain and in the US. With a few notable exceptions, physicians generally have been less than enthusiastic about the therapeutic indications for selenium, probably because they do not understand them.

This is, to my mind, an unfortunate state of affairs and quite a worrying one because, as Dr Gunther Tolg, one of the world's most respected and venerated organic chemists, reported in 1984 from the Max-Planck Institute in Stuttgart, as a result of exhaustive research using the most sophisticated techniques, a significant trend towards lower selenium intake throughout the world has been confirmed. So not only are the health protective advantages of selenium still being overlooked, but selenium intakes are diminishing due to natural causes. It is my hope, therefore, that further medical research will be conducted into selenium as a prophylactic agent.

There is no cause for medical complacency in the face of the major killing and disabling diseases. Even in civilized western countries with sophisticated medical services, it is obvious to all with the will to look that the overall picture is grim. Rheumatism, in all its forms, still cripples and maims countless thousands, and the impact of modern rheumatology has made only small inroads into this massive arena of suffering. Despite enormous efforts on behalf of sufferers from arteriosclerotic heart disease, by both medicine and surgery, we still find ourselves in the middle of a world-wide coronary disease epidemic.

A little while ago it began to look as if, through new methods of chemical and radiological control — together with progress in the field of earlier diagnosis brought about by more sophisticated imaging techniques — we were winning the battle against cancer. Unfortunately, a special article in the world-famous and prestigious American

New England Journal of Medicine that hailed from the Harvard School of Public Health and the University of Iowa Medical Center in 1986 lowered all our hopes on this score too.

This study assessed the overall progress against cancer from 1950 to 1982 in the US. These years, it demonstrated, were associated with *increases* in the crude cancer-related mortality rate, and *increases* in the age-adjusted mortality rate, and in both the crude and age-adjusted incidence rates. The only bright spark on the horizon in this comprehensive study was that survival times for cancer victims became rather longer. Understandably, the authors of this careful survey concluded that we are losing the war against cancer. They advocate a shift in research emphasis — a shift from research on treatment to research on prevention. That selenium seems capable of playing an enormous part in that prevention remains largely ignored.

But, as well as areas of well-documented, if little heeded, evidence of selenium being a unique health prophylactic in three of the major disease areas (rheumatism, heart disease and cancer), there is other preliminary evidence of further health advantages that may well derive from the intelligent use of this micronutrient.

———— Radiation hazards and selenium ————

The recent tragic and worrying Russian atomic energy accident at Chernobyl re-alerted the world to how potentially vulnerable we all are to accidents leading to radiation disease. It will be years before the full toll of loss of life from delayed neoplastic disease (cancers) can be calculated from this one incident alone.

In the United States the accident that occurred at the nuclear energy plant on Three Mile Island near Harrisburg, Pennsylvania, in 1979 drew wide attention to the dangers of living near a reactor of this sort, and those who live near nuclear plants like Sellafield that seem to be in some way 'accident prone' are understandably anxious on this score. Dr Richard Passwater, whose fame and experience as a 'selenium watcher' has been repeatedly noted elsewhere in this book, has put together his own radiation hazard protection kit. I must admit, if I lived or worked in or near a nuclear energy establishment, I would certainly feel tempted to produce something similar. It would, of course, include kelp or potassium iodide tablets. But it would also include a supply of anti-oxidants, including vitamins A, C, E and selenium.

The evidence that supports such advice is in no way flimsy.

Drs Shimazu and Tappel were drawing attention in *Radiation Research* over twenty years ago to the fact that radiation protection is best effected by molecules that can release or accept electrons and hydrogen atoms, without themselves becoming dissociated. They pointed to selenium compounds — notably seleno-amino acids — as being powerful radiation protectors. This theory was subsequently endorsed by Dr Colonbetti of Pisa and some ten years later by Dr Badiello of the University of Bologna whose work was also reduplicated at the Institute of Cancer Research in Sutton, England.

Although there has been little work on the protective effect against radiation sickness in humans, experiments from the Institute of Internal Medicine at the Medical Academy of Krakow in Poland has demonstrated that mice reared on a selenium-fortified diet survived toxic levels of radiation far better than did similar animals not given supplementary selenium.

——Cystic fibrosis — experimental treatment——

Cystic fibrosis is an example of a disease that we know an awful lot about but in which we can offer little in the way of effective treatment to victims. It is a severe genetic disorder characterized by the body's production of an abnormally 'sticky' mucus and one which produces distressing symptoms involving the lungs, the pancreas and the gastrointestinal tract. It is also, and curiously, associated with increases in the amount of salt in the sweat. This latter characteristic provides a valuable diagnostic test for the disease. From the point of view of heredity, cystic fibrosis is inherited as an autosomal recessive characteristic. This means that the parents of a victim are normally unaffected but one quarter of their children are likely to be born with the disease. Cystic fibrosis is inherited in approximately 1 in 2,000 live births in whites and more rarely in blacks. It is virtually unheard of in oriental populations.

Because the pancreas is affected in cystic fibrosis victims the digestive secretions of this organ are upset and the affected children have difficulty digesting and absorbing fats from their diet. Thick sticky mucus in the respiratory tract also produces wheezy bronchitis, poor respiratory air exchange and predisposes towards chronic chest infection. Unfortunately, apart from energetically treating chest infections as they develop in children with cystic fibrosis and providing them with mechanical aids that help to shift thick and tacky mucus from the chest, there is little that can be done to help the cystic fibrosis victims.

Dr Joel Wallock, as a result of a unique knowledge of comparative pathology (the study of the disease changes in animal tissues in comparison with changes noted in human disease), noted a close similarity between the organs of selenium- and zinc-deficient animals and those of cystic fibrosis victims. He also looked closely at the obstetric history of 15 mothers whose children were born suffering from cystic fibrosis. One thing that he noted was that those mothers who bore cystic fibrosis victims had certain similar characteristics as far as their pregnancies were concerned. All the women involved had less than ideal dietary habits. In 8 of 48 pregnancies the women noticed hair loss or change in hair character during their pregnancy, and there was a relatively high incidence of the disease known as pre-eclampsia (pregnancy toxaemia).

Dr Wallock next set to work on examining the blood of children with cystic fibrosis for selenium and found this to be lower than that of normal children. In two children who had died of cystic fibrosis the blood selenium was at a level of only a tenth of the expected value.

What does all this amount to? Well, on the face of it, not very much. Malabsorption is part and parcel of cystic fibrosis and we must assume that pancreatic deficiency associated with the disease resulted in poor selenium absorption. In other words the selenium deficiency came about as a *result* of the disease rather than being in any way the *cause*. Nevertheless, Dr Wallock showed that in a series of 50 cystic fibrosis cases a special diet free of vegetable oils and with selenium supplementations of between 25 to 300 micrograms of selenium per day brought about quite startling improvements in cystic fibrosis symptomatology including reduced lung mucus, increased energy, improved skin and hair quality, weight gain, increased resistance to infection and reduced secondary signs of respiratory distress.

Subsequent work on selenium and cystic fibrosis has not been particularly encouraging, although there have been several reports of improvement in cystic fibrosis occurring in patients when selenium supplementation of diet has been effected. Most of this work has been done at the Children's Lung Association clinic run by Dr R. F. Goddard at Albuqueque, New Mexico, and at the Cystic Fibrosis Clinic at the University of Miami School of Medicine.

In conclusion it would seem that there is only a remote possibility of altering the liability of a child being born with cystic fibrosis to a carrier woman by manipulation of her antenatal care with selenium or other anti-oxidant substances, for the genetic die is obviously cast at this stage. Nevertheless, as far as the management of the cystic fibrosis victim is concerned, in the face of the lack of any other nutritional or dietary regimen that seems to be otherwise useful a high selenium intake does seem to be a very reasonable way to proceed.

──────Selenium and sexual functioning──────

When I was very much involved in the study of the history of rejuvenation (see Chapter 5), it became obvious to me that as well as the 'life extension' side of rejuvenation the main interest was very closely tied up with sexual rejuvenation and infertility. As there is a deal of confusion on this score perhaps a few definitions are not out of place.

Infertility is easiest to define, so we will deal with this first. Infertility is involved with a *couple's* inability to produce offspring. The basic defect is usually *mostly* related to one member of the union. Most infertility is, however, a *relative and composite* condition. In other words a very fertile man may be able to overcome his partner's diminished fertility and produce a child — and vice versa. Fertility is usually nothing directly to do with sexual potency — an ability to carry out the act of sexual intercourse — although even here the boundaries tend to get rather smudged. (For example, a man who is completely impotent with woman A will be unable to impregnate her, so the fertility in this union is zero. He may, however, be potent and therefore fertile with woman B.)

Sexual potency is related to sexual performance. Men are said to be potent or impotent, but potency can be relative, too. Women are not said to be potent or impotent. If she cannot function satisfactorily sexually, a woman is said to be frigid. Today, doctors do not like to use this perjorative term, and a more modern way to describe her is to say she is sexually dysfunctional. Perhaps one day the term impotence will be dropped, too, and 'male sexual dysfunction' or 'erectile failure' will be used instead of impotence. For to label a man as impotent passes a judgement on him that exceeds his sexual capability in many cases.

The facts of the matter with regard to selenium and infertility are more precise than they are for sexual functioning. Dr U. M. Cowgill of the University of Pittsburgh has looked at the medical geography of selenium through the publications of the National Center for Health Statistics and Population data that are used in the production of the US census. They showed that there is a higher birth rate in high soil and high crop selenium areas than in medium or low selenium areas. Low selenium areas also have a higher infant mortality.

Animal experiments have proved that profound selenium deficiency produces infertile animals. The basic cause of the infertility in these cases seems to lie in the male reproductive contribution to the union, and male animals reared on a selenium-deficient diet produce few sperm cells, and those that are produced function poorly. Sheep breeders in New Zealand (a land hampered in many ways by low soil selenium) find that there is a great improvement in fertility if the sheep's diet is supplemented by selenium. Work at Oregon State University has also shown that selenium deficiency adversely effects the sperm quality in rats, and an interesting sidelight to this research is that radioactive (labelled) selenium seems to 'home in' on the testes and 25-40 per cent of it finishes up in the male sex organs.

There seems to have been little work carried out on the specific effects of selenium on the female germ cells (the ova or eggs) probably because experimental work in this whole area is simpler and cheaper in the male than in the female.

Exactly where we are with relation to the infertile union and selenium would seem to be that selenium deficiency is very definitely related to lowered fertility and that, when infertility is related to low soil selenium, selenium supplementation of the diet improves fertility. In all probability, whether or not a man, or a woman, is getting enough selenium to maintain a high state of fertility depends on two things — the amount of selenium in the foods swallowed and the efficiency of the absorption organ to extract selenium from the food. It is possible to get a fair idea of whether or not you live in a selenium-rich or -poor area, but to find out about your absorption organ's efficiency is very much more difficult — if not impossible, and so once again selenium supplements may solve the problem.

———— Selenium and sexual performance ————

The more that scientists and physicians ponder about the whole subject of sexual functioning, the more confused the whole problem seems to become. One of the reasons for this is that new knowledge has led to new thinking on this score. When, over a decade ago, Dr William Masters and his co-workers were publishing their original work on sexual functioning, they claimed that 90 per cent of all sexual dysfunction (impotence and frigidity) was psychological as far as causation was concerned. But, over the years, careful and painstaking research has shown this not to be a true statement of the position. Now, even the doyens of the world of sex therapy who, of course, treat their patients by psychological methods, are tending to agree with medical research that suggests that at least 30 per cent of sexual dysfunction, in both sexes, is due to physical rather than psychological causes, and that all the psychological sex therapy in the world is unlikely to benefit this unfortunate group of men and women.

When this so-called organic sexual dysfunction is examined in more detail, two major disease states appear to be involved, diabetes and occlusive arterial disease (the old friend we met in Chapter 7). Again, most of the experimental and therapeutic work has been carried out on sexually dysfunctional men (impotent or erectile failure victims). Research carried out mostly in continental Europe has identified a group of such men that have severe arteriosclerotic defects in the arteries that supply blood to the penis. It would seem likely that these changes are identical to those that affect the coronary arteries in anginal victims.

One very fashionable way to treat the severe angina victim, or the person whose severe arterial disease is threatening the efficiency of his whole heart muscle, is to offer 'by-pass' surgery in which various branches of severely diseased artery are replaced by a healthy vessel. In many cases such operations give new lives to patients. Men whose pelvic arteries are producing erectile failure and subsequent impotence are often operated upon in European centres and are given pelvic artery by-pass surgery. Success of this form of surgical treatment is affirmed by results. It is far from uncommon for the patient to 'come around' from his operation with an erection!

It has always seemed strange to me how much we ignore quite startling evidence in the field of preventative medicine. The smoker will often ignore the effects of nicotine on his arteries until angina strikes or intermittent claudication produces such a pain in his calf muscle that he cannot walk another step without a pause to rest. There is a mass of evidence that selenium supplementation and a regular ration of marine oil in place of animal fat in our diet is arterio-protective as far as cardiovascular disease is concerned. It would be quite extraordinary if it did not have a similar protective effect on pelvic arterial disease and sexual potency too.

Is there any evidence that selenium therapy is helpful in the case of the 70 per cent majority of folk of both sexes who run into problems of sexual dysfunction on psychological grounds? Richard Passwater believes that there is and argues that the greatest aphrodisiac is good health and abundant energy. Klaus Schwartz, a man who is remembered as the father of selenium, noted that one of the first signs of selenium deficiency is an impairment of mitochondrial functioning. The mitochondria are the vital components in cells that mobilize energy synthesis. The free radicals that we met in Chapter 5 are particularly toxic to mitochondria, and we do know that selenium rates high among the anti-oxidants that have an enviable reputation as far as protection against free radical damage is concerned.

The exact contribution that inadequate selenium intake or absorption makes to the whole subject of sexual dysfunction remains *sub judice* at the moment. Many of us have a hunch that it could be considerable.

CHAPTER 12
Selenium as health insurance

In many ways we are just beginning to appreciate the real importance of the trace elements and minerals as far as our health and general welfare are concerned. Hopefully this book has 'got you going' in this matter, and pointed you in the right direction so that you and yours can be both on the lookout for possible health hazards that are associated with trace element deprivation in general and selenium lack in particular. Hopefully, too, it has pushed the gates of the new nutritional knowledge open far enough for you to peep in and have a look around and see what selenium can do for you in the matter of life extension. Really this 'live long and stay young' message is clearer now than it has ever been.

Getting down to practical matters

Practicality is the essence of all effective health education — especially where health education leans heavily on nutritional science. The practicality of making sure you get enough selenium in your food to confirm that your health insurance premiums are fully paid up is very important if trace element health dividends and bonuses are to be gained regularly. Answers to the following questions must be found and acted upon. First of all, who needs selenium supplementation? Secondly, how can we modify our eating habits to improve our selenium intake? Finally, if selenium supplementation is necessary then what form should it take and how much should we take and for how long?

Who needs selenium supplementation?

As we have seen in Chapter 4 it depends to some extent on medical geography and where you live. In the United States, research carried out by G. Schrauzer and by the USDA Technical Bulletin staff have produced some interesting 'selenium maps' that indicate the highs and lows of soil selenium and, as we have seen, the relationship between these areas and the incidence of certain diseases. In Britain, although similar evidence is not available in such detail, an interesting and valuable survey was carried out by a couple of scientists from the Ministry of Agriculture, Fisheries and Food in 1977 in conjunction with N. G. Bunton from the Laboratory of the Government Chemist. This was a very practical exercise in which personnel from a group of selected colleges in the United Kingdom went out shopping to buy some 80 major foodstuffs, appropriate to their location and time of year, and then prepared them for the table and analysed the selenium they contained. The areas involved were Cardiff (Wales), Edinburgh (Scotland) and Shrewsbury, Newcastle, Uxbridge and London. Food selection was made both with reference to providing a fair mixed diet, and to items that might be expected to be rich and low in selenium. Each food sample was analysed by a standard method known to give a 95 per cent confidence limit.

Unfortunately, owing to variations in sampling, washing, preparing and cooking the various foods, it was not possible to give regional values for food selenium content in this study and so the results obtained reflect a mean value for UK cities.

It was obvious from this research that the richest source of selenium in British food is fish. But so little fish is eaten in the UK today that it only makes a relatively small contribution to our total selenium intake and we get most of our selenium from cereals. It was also noted in this report that our estimated intake of selenium averaged only 60 micrograms daily. Quite obviously many of our population take much less than this because substantial areas of Britain are known to have a low soil, and therefore crop, selenium. Modern scientific opinion inclines to the view that a daily intake of at least 200 micrograms of selenium should be taken to maintain optimum health.

It is pretty obvious that most of the population of Britain fell short on selenium (with the notable East Anglian exceptions). In other words, we all need more selenium.

Eating better for selenium

Clearly, if we look at any list of foods that shows relative selenium content it is possible to spot 'best buys' in the selenium market place. But, even so, there are pitfalls for the unwary to fall into if you are not careful. Fish looks and is a good source of selenium. It also has an excellent track record as far as being cardio-protective on the grounds of its marine oil content as we saw in Chapter 7. Many authorities, however, point out that due to the way selenium is conjugated in fish with other elemental substances, only a small proportion of the selenium in fish is actually absorbed into our body, and so eating more fish, although providing a health bonus in other ways, will not solve the nation's selenium deficiency.

Another way to get more selenium into our systems would be to increase our daily intake of cereals. But, here again, there are potential and actual problems. The selenium in cereals is very much influenced by geography.

The flour that is mostly used by the bread-making industry comes largely from North American sources and has a relatively high selenium content. But the modern vogue is for 'home baked' special breads like wholemeal and other high-fibre breads often involving 'home grown' cereals. This tendency, the Ministry of Agriculture scientists point out, means much less selenium is taken in our cereal food. When we look to other cereal sources in this country: pastas, rice, porridge oats and breakfast cereals in general, these the Ministry analyst has found to be 'among the lowest in the literature'. No explanation of this curious state of affairs has been given. But it would seem likely that the heat and chemical processing of breakfast cereal manufacture probably profoundly reduces its selenium content.

Meat as a source of selenium 'looks good' on most lists and does provide the major selenium contribution to the British way of life — kidney being a particularly rich source. It is interesting, however, that the Ministry of Agriculture survey found that the selenium content of carcass meat and offal (and, incidentally, fish) was lower than in most USA reports. Why was this? The reasons are not obvious, but they may indicate that some selenium depletion occurs when food is 'collected' by normal shopping techniques and then is cooked for consumption (as opposed to food delivered to laboratories for scientific analysis where it may well be analysed raw or without the various processes undertaken by domestic cooking and preparation).

It is incredible how quickly almost any subject develops its own 'folklore', and selenium is no exception to this. Garlic and mushrooms are traditionally accepted as being selenium-rich foods. But, as far as mushrooms are concerned, the type of mushroom and the composition of the mushroom compost it is grown on alters the selenium content significantly, as does the cooking technique. The Ministry of Agriculture confirmed that both of these relatively rare items of diet contained some selenium but in 'lower quantities than reported elsewhere'. In case you come to the conclusion that the government chemists involved in this study were just not very good at detecting selenium in the food they sampled, when they got around to analysing the selenium in nuts — including brazil nuts, peanuts, cashew nuts and walnuts — they found rather higher values than 'reported elsewhere'. Perhaps the worst news for potential selenium eaters, however, came from the Ministry's analysis of British vegetables generally and milk in particular. These were below the level of detection of selenium!

Our drinking water in Britain contains no selenium, and so popular British drinks and beverages are virtually selenium-free too. Mother's milk and baby foods are very low in selenium and it is not until cereals are introduced into the diet of young children that they get their first 'top-up' of selenium — until this happy day they have to 'make do' with the selenium they are born with.

All in all it would seem that unless meat and offal are eaten in quantity and regularly, and cereal from North American sources is freely available and taken in substantial quantities, 'eating for selenium' is something of a lost cause, and that if we want to be quite sure we get enough selenium to enjoy its potential health benefits then dietary supplementation seems to be the only practical proposition in the UK, as is indeed the case as far as iodine is concerned.

How much and which sort — and for how long?

It would be really nice if we could get all the selenium we need the natural way — through our food. In Finland, as previously mentioned, the authorities are trying to replace the selenium in their depleted soil so as to improve the selenium content of their grain. But it looks as though this is a long and expensive process. Clearly, a greater use of raw unprocessed cereal food would help natural dietary intake, and perhaps microwave cooking might improve the ultimate 'on the plate' content of selenium in our food, too.

Regular, preferably daily, dietary supplementation is, however, at the moment going to be the most practical way of gaining health insurance from selenium for all and sundry, and particularly those for whom absorption problems exist that hamper the absorption of trace elements. Within this probably substantial group are the elderly, the very young, those who self-select special diets (particularly low calorie slimming diets), vegans and the enormous group of 'idiopathic' poor absorbers. These are folk whom we can detect only through the symptomology of selenium depletion and will probably be rheumatism sufferers, those with chronic arterial disease or certain cancer victims.

In all probability the 'how much?' problem has been solved and the Food and Nutrition Board's 1977 resolution of 200 micrograms per day has now been given world-wide acceptance. On the question of 'how long?', little is known about selenium storage and the various factors that tend to antagonize selenium absorption. Unfortunately, tests for selenium in the body are both expensive and generally unobtainable so the most sensible way to look at selenium dosage is to treat selenium like any other vital nutrient and take it daily.

The many forms of selenium

Selenium, we must remember, is basically an element that occurs in food as are carbon, nitrogen and oxygen. But, like these constituents of our food, it does not occur in elemental form in Nature but as complex molecules and in packages of molecules. Different foods contain different packages of their vital elements. For instance, proteins all contain some nitrogen, whereas refined carbohydrates and fats contain mostly carbon, oxygen and hydrogen. Rarely, when there is a deficiency of a trace element in the diet that is causing disease processes (like iodine deficiency causing goitre) is it possible to cure or prevent the problem just by giving the element (or a salt of the element) concerned (like adding iodine to table salt). There is evidence that a selenium salt, sodium selenite, which is used mostly in veterinary work — prevents the selenium deficiency diseases in certain animals. But 'organic' selenium holds pride of place in the whole complex spectrum of selenium supplementation as far as humans are concerned.

The selenium in our food is naturally enough 'organic' (mostly in the form of what organic chemists call seleno-amino acids). Let's call it 'selenium protein'. But, even so, not all selenium protein forms are equal as far as selenium assimilation is concerned, even though they are much better than simple inorganic selenium compounds like selenium dioxide (an inorganic selenium compound that even if given in high dosage fails to raise blood levels of selenium very much). Dr Klaus Schwartz (the man with the dream that came true) is said to have synthesized 800 organic selenium compounds, most of which, instead of circulating in the blood and doing good, tended to get deposited in fat and thus effectively removed from the circulation.

Eventually a form of organic selenium (selenium yeast) was elaborated by Dr Gerhard Schrauzer, of the University of California in San Diego, who carried out tests on natural organically bound selenium in brewer's yeast and found that this form of selenium protein was twenty times more effective than inorganic selenium in building up blood selenium levels.

Yeast is of course a 'health food' of some antiquity. Taken at one time as a potent source of vitamin B it was often prescribed for patients who were 'run down', particularly if they suffered from boils or acne. Brewer's yeast contains some selenium, but in the early 1970s it was discovered that when yeasts are raised in a medium containing inorganic selenium salts then selenium in appreciable amounts becomes incorporated into the yeast. From the biochemical point of view the selenium replaces the element sulphur in the sulphur-containing proteins of some plants, including yeasts. What happens is that an element, i.e. selenium, becomes part of a food — yeast is, for all intents and purposes, a vegetable food.

By now the whole subject of selenium absorption from selenium yeast has been extensively studied and all reports favour an organic (yeast) selenium supplement fortified with vitamins A, C and E as the compound of choice.

Finale

This book was written to bring to as wide an audience as possible the present state of knowledge as far as selenium is concerned. In no way was it our intention to pass selenium off as a panacea for all the ills that human flesh is heir to. To some extent that task is difficult because selenium works in the tissues at a cellular and subcellular level, acting upon the very working parts of our cells — their *organelles*. Klaus Schwartz's 'dream' to be responsible for the eradication of one disease that plagues mankind has been seen to come true with selenium. But much more research is necessary before we can fully understand intercellular physiology and before we can explain *why* the dream came true and how we can best harness our new knowledge to make other diseases and disabilities a bad dream of our time. But much more than just a germ of an idea is with us now.

Index

absorption, 24-5; organ, 68-74, 85, 91
acid rain, 30, 31-2
ageing: controlled, 38-40; planned, 37; random, 37
agriculture: remedies in, 9-10; selenium in, 65-6
alternative medicine, 75-6
anaemia, 13, 15
angina, 16, 51, 55, 86
anti-oxidants, 67, 81, 87; and rheumatism, 45; and random ageing, 39, 40
arteries: disease of, 51-4, 86, 92
atheromatous disease, 51
atherosclerosis, 51, 53, 55, 67, 80
arthritis, 43, 45-6, 47; and selenium, 15, 22, 41-7; see also osteo-arthritis
auto-immune disease, 44, 77

bio-availability: of selenium, 73-4
blood selenium levels, 58-60, 61, 62, 78-9
bowel dysfunction, 71
British Medical Journal, BMJ: and cancer study, 62-3

cancer, 56-7, 59, 60, 61, 67, 80-1, 92; and nutrition, 36; and selenium, 29, 56-66
cereals, 31, 32, 33, 60, 65, 73, 90, 91
chemicals: and cancer, 56
China: heart disease in, 39; Keshan disease in, 48-9
cocoa workers: and malaria, 30-1
cod liver oil: and rheumatism, 21
cold syndrome, 74-5
concentration gradient system, 71
coronary heart disease, 8, 26, 30, 51, 52, 54, 80; and selenium, 48-55
cross linking: and ageing, 40, 68
cures: testimonials for, 18-22
cystic fibrosis, 82-4

deficiency disease, 13, 17, 30; ecology, 30-1; maps, 29-30; auto-immune, 44
diet, 68, 83, 88; and cancer, 57, 60, 63, 64; and Keshan disease, 50; and longevity, 35, 36; and selenium, 72-4
dietary supplement, of selenium, 16, 40, 45, 49-50, 72-74, 83-4, 88-93; and cancer, 58, 64, 65; and infertility, 85
dosage: of selenium, 91-2

East Anglia: and soil selenium, 7, 8, 9, 37, 65, 89
Ecuador: longevity in, 35
enzymes, 13; and ageing, 39

fenugreek, 10
Finland, 60, 61, 62, 65-6

Index

fish, 32, 51, 52, 89; as selenium source, 27-8, 31, 33, 52, 73, 89-90
food: local, 9, 37, 72; and medical geography, 33, 89; and selenium, 24, 26, 28, 35-6, 63, 69-70, 73
free radicals, 37, 38, 45, 47, 54, 67, 68, 87

genetics, 25, 39, 56
glutathione peroxidase, 13, 39, 45
goitres, 13, 68-9
gout, 33, 41

hartnup disease, 69
health, 9, 10, 12-13, 88
heart disease, 48-55
herbs, 9, 20
hormones, 44; and HRT, 21

IBS, irritable bowel syndrome, 71
immune system, 77-9
infertility, 84-5
iodine, 13, 68-9
iron, 13, 15, 16, 19, 76-7

joints, 42, 43, 67

Keshan disease, 48-50

Legionnaire's disease, 79
life: healthier, 9; longevity of, 7-9, 35-40

lymphocytes, 77-8

malaria, 30, 31
malnutrition, 30
mandrake plant, 9
maps: and disease, 29-30, 88
meat: selenium in, 33, 63-4, 74, 90
medical geography, 29-34, 49-50, 51, 58, 88
menopause, 16, 20-1, 38
minerals, 10, 13, 23, 26, 88
mushrooms, 73-4, 90

nervous system, 17
New Zealand: and muscle weakness, 39-40
NSAID, non-steroidal anti-inflammatory drugs, 42
nutrients, 13, 22, 23, 24-5, 76; micro, 67, 80
nutrition: science of, 23
nuts: selenium in, 91

oestrogen: and herbs, 20, 21
orchid, purple, 9
'organic' selenium, 92-3
osteoarthritis, 41, 42, 47
overweight: and nutrition, 26
oxygen: in ageing, 38; and free radicals, 38, 39

Pakistan: and longevity, 35, 36
Passwater, Dr Richard, 13, 29, 45, 54, 81, 86
penicillamine, 44, 45
physiotherapy, 42, 44
placebo response, 18, 19, 20, 46
preventative medicine, 86
progeria, 39
prophylactic agent, 80
prostaglandins, 54-5
psychology: and ill-health, 76; and sexual dysfunction, 85
psychotrophic effect: of trace elements, 16-17

radiation: and selenium, 81-2
RDA, Recommended Daily Allowance, 23-4, 26, 33
rheumatic fever, 51
rheumatism, 21, 41, 43-5, 46, 80, 92; and free radicals, 45, 67; and selenium, 14-15, 16, 21, 22, 41-7
rubber plantations: and malaria, 31
'run-down' syndrome, 76

Schwartz, Klaus, 12, 13, 87, 92, 93; and Keshan disease, 48, 50
scurvy, 14, 71-2
selenium absorption,

13, 61, 63, 71, 91; deficiency of, 13, 15, 83, 88; forms of, 92-3; properties of, 9-12; slow action of, 15, 22
sexual functioning, 84-7
smoking: and cancer, 56, 63; and heart disease, 51, 86
soil selenium levels, 8, 29, 30, 36, 37; and acid rain, 31, 32; and cancer, 29, 36, 58, 62; decline in, 32; and infertility, 84-5; maps of, 31, 88; in China, 49-50; in Finland, 62-3, 65, 66; in USA, 54
sources of selenium, 27-8, 33-4, 52, 89-93
stress, 72
synovial membrane, 42, 43, 44, 47, 67

testimonials, 18-22
trace elements, 10-12, 14-16, 23-8, 48, 88; absorption, 71, 72; and bio-availability, 73-4

ulcers, 16
uric acid, 33
USA: selenium levels, 54
uses: of selenium, 14-15
USSR: and longevity, 35, 36

vegetarians: and iron, 77
vitamins, 12-13, 23, 25, 26, 40, 46, 67, 68, 77, 78; and cancer, 59-60, 63, 64; 'A', 63; 'C', 14, 25, 71-2; 'E', 25, 45, 47, 55

Whipple's disease, 69
white cells, 47

yeast: and selenium, 93

zinc, 61